CU00702547

COMMO
GUIDE TO SEX

A COMMONSENSE GUIDE TO SEX

Sandra Pertot
B.A.(Hons), M.Psychol, Ph.D.

ANGUS
& ROBERTSON
PUBLISHERS

ANGUS & ROBERTSON PUBLISHERS

Unit 4, Eden Park, 31 Waterloo Road,
North Ryde, NSW, Australia 2113, and
16 Golden Square, London W1R 4BN,
United Kingdom

First published in Australia
by Angus & Robertson Publishers in 1985
First published in the United Kingdom
by Angus & Robertson (UK) in 1985
Reprinted 1987, 1988

National Library of Australia
Cataloguing-in-publication data

Pertot, Sandra.
　A commonsense guide to sex.

　Bibliography.
　Includes index.
　ISBN 0 207 15151 2.
　ISBN 0 207 15043 5 (pbk).

　1. Sex. I. Title.

612'.6

Typeset in 12pt Garamond by Setrite Typesetters
Printed in Singapore

To Rudi,
Jane and Simon

ACKNOWLEDGEMENTS

I am indebted to Dr J. S. Taylor, urologist, for his help with Chapter 2, and Ray Dorling, clinical psychologist, for his assistance with Chapter 9.

As the ideas expressed in this book have developed over more than a decade of clinical practice and research, it is impossible to identify the original source of many of the ideas discussed. I would like to say, however, that I am particularly grateful to the hundreds of men and women who have trusted me enough to confide in me about their sex lives.

CONTENTS

INTRODUCTION

NOT ANOTHER BOOK ABOUT SEX!

I am sure that is the reaction of many when they first pick up this book. Surely it has all been said before? Sex must account for more books and articles than any other topic. What makes me think I could possibly have anything new to say on the subject?

In my work over the last decade as a clinical psychologist, I have specialised in the treatment of sexual problems. Because of this I have made a point of reading as much of the available literature on sex as possible, so that I would be able to recommend helpful books and articles to my clients. Yet I found that there were very few I would recommend with confidence.

Why?

Because most of these books are either moralistic, sensational, unrealistic, boring or just plain wrong.

The moralists tell us what is supposed to be right or wrong, the sensationalists describe sex as an overwhelming, mind-blowing experience. Others raise unrealistic expectations about sex, implying that it should always be enjoyable and satisfying, no matter what else might be happening in your life at that time. Some books go into infinite detail, with pages and pages of step-by-step instructions about every aspect of sexuality. Still others give out damaging

1

false information, such as the book that claimed that any woman who does not enjoy sex has a serious psychological problem.

Most books, despite the disclaimers of their authors, try to impose a stereotype on sexual behaviour. One book went to great lengths to talk about every woman's individual sexuality, yet said that all women should be able to reach 101 orgasms whenever they have sex. If men ejaculate quickly, or occasionally have problems with erection, or if women find they do not often feel like sex or have difficulty coming to orgasm, this is said to be a SEXUAL PROBLEM and something needs to be done about it.

These books tend to make people feel inadequate, rather than encouraging them to feel more confident about the way they are conducting their sexual relationships.

What is the missing ingredient?

COMMONSENSE!

Commonsense involves the recognition that sex is not always a magical experience that is exciting and enjoyable, no matter what. Commonsense suggests that people are different, and want and need different things from sex. Commonsense means that it is normal for people to sometimes find sex boring, or at times to feel resentful, angry, irritated or annoyed by the thought or act of sex.

Sexual expression takes many forms in different people, and often even in the same person at different times in his or her life. No-one can say what is right for all people. What people believe to be appropriate sexual behaviour depends on such factors as culture, religion and family background. There is no definitive set of attitudes or behaviours that can or should apply to all people everywhere.

This means that no single book is going to have all the answers for all people. Some who read this book might find it boring, some might find it disgusting, some may simply find it irrelevant because their particular problem is not discussed. Others, hopefully, will find it a welcome relief to learn that they are not so different after all.

I would therefore encourage readers to read critically. Take from the book what is useful or appropriate, and ignore the rest. Have confidence in your own judgement to disagree with anything that does not apply to you.

The aim of this book is for you to learn about your own sexuality, and gain confidence in your own judgement about your sexual needs and desires. It is not a "how-to-do-it" book in the sense that it goes into detail about different sexual techniques and positions. This is covered more than adequately in countless other books. It is aimed at the couple who have a commitment to a long-term relationship, and who would like to feel more comfortable with their sex life.

The underlying philosophy of this book is that, with a bit of commonsense, you can take charge of your own sexuality so that you can develop the type of sexual relationship you find enjoyable.

1 WHAT WE LEARN ABOUT SEX FROM OUR SOCIETY

In this book I am hoping to explore sexuality from a commonsense standpoint, and to be as objective and practical as possible.

Sometimes, however, this approach leads to criticism, because some people believe it is degrading sex, belittling its importance and beauty. Some believe that many of the practical suggestions given are perverted or abnormal. Others see them as immoral or sinful.

We need to recognise that sex is very much like politics and religion. What we believe about these things depends on how, when and where we were brought up. By this I mean that our ideas about sexuality are tremendously influenced by our family, our friends, our schools, the media; in short, by the society in which we live.

This point can be appreciated when we look at the sexual attitudes and behaviours found in other societies. By doing this it is possible to come to the realisation that many of the ideas we cherish with regard to sex may not be so absolutely right as we have always thought.

This is not to say that we must then necessarily change our ideas. We all need a set of values and beliefs to help us make decisions about our lives. Also, it is very difficult to suddenly change and accept something that we might have thought of as wrong for many years. Hopefully, though, we will come to understand our own feelings and behaviours more clearly, and in doing so, become less anxious about ourselves. Along the way we may also become more tolerant of others who think and behave differently.

OTHER SOCIETIES

No society is completely homogeneous. That is, in any one society, individuals with different points of view about almost any topic can be found. For example, although the Roman Empire became known for its permissive attitude to sex, records have been found of prominent citizens deploring the trend toward promiscuity and the disregard of tradition.

With this in mind, we will take a brief look at some of the fascinating differences in the sexual practices of various societies throughout history.

Marriage

In western society, we tend to practise monogamous marriage, which means one wife for one husband. In recent years, there has been increasing acceptance of serial monogamy, that is, ending one monogamous relationship before entering into another.

Many societies, however, have practised polygamous marriage. The most common form of this is polygyny, whereby one husband takes several wives. Polygyny dates back to ancient times and often came about for practical reasons. Frequent wars often caused a shortage of men, so a plurality of wives was a practical way of looking after the surplus of women. Also, because it took time to bring a child into the world, polygyny made it possible for one man to make several women pregnant at the same time and thus increase the population of the tribe. In the recent past, polygyny took on a religious meaning when it was sanctioned, for a brief time, by the American Mormons.

Less common is the practice of polyandry, where one woman took more than one husband at a time. The most obvious reason for this custom was a situation in which men outnumbered women. This was common among races which extensively practised female infanticide. Other reasons included poverty on the part of the man, when he could not afford to acquire and keep a full-time wife.

Premarital sex

Premarital sex still is a contentious issue in our society, despite rapidly changing attitudes. Twenty years ago it was definitely regarded as immoral, although research suggests that what people believed and what they really did were two different things. Studies by Kinsey and his colleagues in America in the late 1940s found that despite the prevailing negative attitude to premarital sex, 83 per cent of males and 50 per cent of females were reported to have experienced intercourse premaritally. Now the figures are likely to be over 90 per cent for both sexes, for young people currently marrying.

Premarital sex in some societies has been regarded as normal and even encouraged. Some societies, such as the Trobriand Islanders, provided mixed houses for single males and females. In some communities, premarital sex was not meant to lead to marriage; it was thought to be just as natural to spontaneously satisfy sexual needs as to satisfy hunger and thirst. Elsewhere, it was regarded as a method of courtship by trial and error which led gradually to marriage. But there are other societies, such as the Kuku of Sumatra, where sexual intercourse before marriage was not tolerated, and if it occurred the couple was punished in some way. In a number of cultures, proof of virginity of the woman was demanded at marriage.

In many societies, a double standard existed in the attitude towards premarital sex by a male or a female. In ancient Rome, for example, it was unthinkable that a male would wait till marriage before having sex, but a female was seriously disgraced if she were not a virgin at marriage.

Obviously, in communities where chastity was demanded, premarital pregnancy was a disgrace. But even in some societies where premarital sex was permitted, pregnancy was often punished. For example, although the Melanesian communities of New Guinea and the adjacent archipelago allowed full sexual freedom before marriage, the occurrence of a pregnancy under such circumstances was a grave disgrace to the mother, and the child was penalised throughout life. Elsewhere, for a girl to have given birth prior to marriage was a high recommendation, since it was evidence of her fertility.

Extramarital sex

As with premarital sex, sexual relations outside marriage have been regarded throughout history and in diverse cultures in a variety of ways. Contemporary Catholics regard adultery as a mortal sin, whereas a man of the Roman Empire considered it absurd to even contemplate restricting his sexual relations to his wife.

Throughout history, however, adultery by the wife has been regarded far more seriously than adultery by the husband. Some cultures allowed, even encouraged, the enraged husband to execute his wife under these circumstances, while he could have affairs with impunity. Even in recent historical times, for example, in Victorian England, adultery of the man was of no consequence if his lover were unmarried. Adultery of a married woman was different. Since a wife was legally regarded as a possession of her husband, he could take out a civil action against the offending male and get monetary compensation for his wife's loss of virtue.

A more controlled form of extramarital sex is the practice of wife-lending as a form of hospitality. A husband expressed genuine friendship by making available his wife to a visitor. Eskimos practised this custom without shame or horror. A child born of such a union had a special name for its father, speaking of him as "the man who slept with my mother".

Masturbation

The first sexual act most commonly engaged in is self-stimulation, or masturbation. Babies, both male and female as young as a few months old, have been observed stimulating their genitals. They derive obvious pleasure from such actions, even, it seems, achieving some type of orgasm.

As with other sexual behaviours, masturbation has been reviled by some societies and accepted, even encouraged, by others. Indeed, in some primitive cultures, it was quite acceptable for the mother to stimulate her baby's genitals to soothe him, whereas in our society we would regard that as sexual abuse.

The ancient Greeks and Romans viewed masturbation as a healthy safety valve against sexual frustration, for both men and women. The ancient Chinese viewed masturbation as acceptable for women, but not men as it led to the wasting of semen, his source of energy. The Christian Church has always regarded masturbation as a sin. Parents in Victorian England were warned to go to great lengths to stop their children masturbating not only because it was regarded as a sin, but also because it was thought to lead to all sorts of illnesses, even early death.

Enjoyment of sex

It might seem almost absurd to have a section to look at whether people think sex should be enjoyable or not. Yet, like every other aspect of sexuality, there has been, and still is, disagreement over whether sex should be pleasurable, and if so, to what extent.

Initially, primitive humans were totally unaware

of the relationship between sex and procreation, so clearly in our earliest history sex was pursued for physical satisfaction alone.

Even after the connection between intercourse and pregnancy was realised, sex continued to be sought after for pleasure as well as for the begetting of children. Many ancient civilisations, the Romans, the Greeks, the Egyptians, viewed sex as a pleasurable occupation to be pursued with enthusiasm. It is difficult to discover whether women were expected to get as much pleasure from sex as men, or whether men put any emphasis on pleasuring the female as well as themselves. It is clear, though, that women were certainly regarded as having the ability to enjoy sex. However, the double standard that we have previously encountered allowed men much greater freedom in their pursuit of sexual pleasure.

The ancient Chinese, following the philosophy of Taoism, elevated sexual pleasure to a spiritual obligation. Sex was a sacred duty that the Taoist should perform frequently and conscientiously. Basic to the philosophy is the concept of "Yin" and "Yang" which were opposing, yet complementary, forces. "Yin" was the passive feminine force, "Yang" the active masculine force. Intercourse was regarded as the first stage in achieving "Yin-Yang" harmony. Women's "Yin" essence was believed to be inexhaustible, and could nourish the man's "Yang" essence, or semen, which was limited in quantity. "Yang" quality was of extreme importance, and needed to be regularly strengthened by the "Yin" essence during intercourse. Therefore, men were encouraged to have intercourse with as many women as possible, aiming for a goal of 10 women in one night. The ideal, according to detailed Chinese handbooks, was for a man to prolong intercourse for as long as possible; the longer he remained inside, the more "Yin" essence he would absorb. He must also, without fail, rouse her to orgasm, when her essence reached maximum potency. Since his own essence could be depleted by ejaculation, the Taoist aimed at withholding ejaculation indefinitely. However, if he had intercourse with a prostitute, her "Yin" essence was so powerful because she had frequent intercourse with different men, that he could afford to relax and ejaculate without too much loss of "Yang".

At the same time that the Chinese were endowing sex with this great importance for health and happiness, the fathers of the early Christian Church were advocating sexual abstinence as the only sure route to heaven. There was a general feeling among the Church fathers that the act of intercourse was fundamentally disgusting. It was variously regarded as filthy and degrading, unseemly, unclean, shameful and a defilement. Sex was sanctioned only in marriage, and then only for the purpose of procreation. To the Church, sexual pleasure was a sin.

Nineteenth-century England epitomises this attitude to sexuality. Sexual pleasure was frequently regarded as carnal lust, although some writers, such as Elizabeth Blackwell, endowed sex with a righteous spiritualism that lifted sex way above the carnal level. Nevertheless, sex was primarily regarded by middle-class moralists as being only for procreation. It was conceded that men were, unfortunately, the victims of animalistic passion, but women were thought to be "not very much troubled with sexual feeling of any kind". A modest woman submitted to her husband only to please him, not out of any desire for gratification herself. And masturbation was not only sinful, but positively harmful, causing anything from acne to mental illness and ultimately an early death. Sexual pleasure was strictly for the unfortunate few who could not control themselves.

Conclusion

Need we go any further? We could look at other aspects of sexuality such as homosexuality, accepted techniques and positions, and so on, but surely the point is made.

It is impossible to lay down set rules about what is right or wrong sexual behaviour.

Ultimately, you must make your own decisions about what you consider is right for you, and these decisions will be influenced to some degree by what you have learnt about sexuality from our society.

OUR SOCIETY

Western society seems to be in such a state of rapid change, and encompasses such a variety of beliefs, that it is hard to tell whether we are becoming increasingly uninhibited, or whether the sexual revolution has peaked and we are on our way back into a conservative era.

This confusion arises because there are two dominating strands of thought current in our society.

On the one hand, there are the traditionalists,

those who view the current openness towards sexual issues as immoral and sinful. Britain has Mrs Mary Whitehouse and her supporters, the United States has the Moral Majority movement, and Australia has the Reverend Fred Nile and the Festival of Light.

This group says that sex should only take place in marriage, that it is a private event and should not be discussed, and that masturbation and homosexuality, among other things, are perversions. According to them, sex education should be left to the parents who are, supposedly, best able to tell children how beautiful sex is.

On the other hand, we have the sensationalists, the new era of recent decades. This view is most heavily propagated by the media. Some authors, such as Harold Robbins, specialise in super-sexy novels where the characters are always wildly sexual. One female character I recall from one such book was able to reach orgasm walking down the street, merely by squeezing her thighs! Films shown in the cinema are visually not as explicit, although the booming video-recorder trade is making sexually explicit films readily available for private use. The theme is always the same: arousal occurs easily, men perform wondrous feats, and women writhe in enjoyment. Sex is wonderful, enjoyable, can be had anywhere, anytime, with anyone, and anything is permissible because mature, sophisticated people enjoy every-thing.

What do these seemingly diametrically opposed viewpoints have in common?

IGNORANCE!

The first says that sex is love and therefore good

sex will automatically follow if the couple love each other enough. Conversely, if sex is not enjoyable, it must be because their relationship is not good enough. It is not that long ago that a woman who could not come to orgasm was likely to be advised to consider leaving her husband because it meant she did not love him.

According to this approach, sex education centres on this "sex is love" theme, ignoring the need to understand our bodies and how they work. Sex education is regarded as teaching about menstruation and where babies come from. This is biology, not sexuality, and does not help either boy or girl to understand sexual feelings and enjoy them.

Equally as bad, however, is the other viewpoint. This says that sex is easy, no learning required. Automatically both males and females can perform wondrous feats. How embarrassing not to understand all aspects of sexuality, or to have any sexual inhibitions! How immature and unsophisticated! Good heavens, don't tell me you have a sexual hang-up!

The disciples of this line of thinking totally ignore the need to learn how to have an enjoyable sex life. More importantly, they set unrealistic, rigid stereotypes for sexual success. They completely ignore the fact that there is tremendous variability in people's sexual ideas and behaviours. A person's sexuality is as individual as his height, eye colour, sporting interests, fingerprints and food preferences. And they seem to be unaware of the fact that their expectations of sexual performance are based more on fantasy than fact. While it may be nice (perhaps) to be like a character from a Harold Robbins novel, I doubt that many people, myself included, could or should try to emulate them!

Both approaches make people embarrassed to learn about sex. The first because sexual curiosity is thought to be a perversion, the second because it is supposedly a sign of immaturity.

How many people feel comfortable buying a book on sex — not men's magazines, etcetera, but a straightforward sex education book? How did you feel when you went into the bookshop to enquire about this book?

Yet if it was a book on yachting, or cooking, or politics, would you have had the same embarrassed hesitation?

Will you feel comfortable if others see you reading this? Can you discuss the issues raised in this book with your partner, or your friends? I am not suggesting that you should do these things, only trying to point out how we make sex one of the things in life that we are most interested in, yet too inhibited to learn about properly.

A good sex life is like everything else. It takes learning, practice, understanding, and patience — from *both* sexes. Men are not automatically endowed with a greater sexual knowledge than women, and they receive no better sex education.

All this leads me to suggest that the biggest sexual problem we have in our society at present is not frigidity, or impotence, or whatever. It is the unrealistic expectations we have of sex, and our ignorance about normal sexual functioning.

Our immaturity and lack of sophistication is not

that we cannot come to orgasm, or do not like oral sex. It is that we are so readily influenced by other people's ideas without having the confidence to determine our own sexuality.

We need the confidence to separate fantasy from reality. When we see John Wayne shoot 12 baddies with a six-bullet gun, we do not expect to copy that. We know it is ridiculous, yet we enjoy it nevertheless. Yet with sex, people feel inadequate if they cannot perform like the super-lovers they see on the screen or read about in novels.

If a five-year-old yearns for a 15-centimetre moulded plastic toy that was described in the television advertisement as being dynamic and exciting, through the use of special effects, we explain to the child that it won't be like that in real life.

This is what we must do with ourselves with regard to sex!

2 WHAT WE'VE GOT AND HOW IT WORKS

Perhaps it is surprising that, despite the number of books and articles dealing with sex, many people still do not fully understand their bodies. Yet many couples who seek counselling for a sexual problem frequently have only a limited knowledge of their own and their partners' bodies.

In this chapter, I will give a relatively brief description of the physical aspects of sexuality. Those interested in more detail will find a reference list at the end of this book.

The question that must be answered in this chapter is: What do we need to know in order to understand and enjoy our bodies?

THE WOMAN

We are going to start with the female because her body is least understood by both herself and her partner. Unlike the male, her genitals are hidden between her legs, so this makes it more difficult for her to accidentally discover what she has. Also, our society does not encourage young women to feel comfortable about their bodies, and to explore their equipment and how it works.

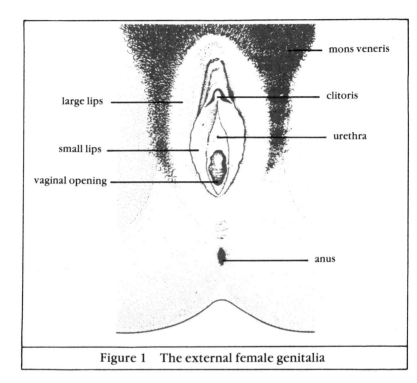

Figure 1   The external female genitalia

Figure 1 gives us a diagrammatic view of the external genitals of the woman, called the *vulva*. First of all, note the Latin name for the pubic area: *mons veneris* or Mount of Venus, who was the Roman goddess of love. What a different attitude to the female genitals from ours today. We tend to think of the genitals as being dirty and smelly, whereas the Romans saw them as the playground for love.

The mons is a pad of fat covering the pubic bone. It is covered with curly hair, and forms the top end of the two *large lips* which protect the genitalia. Like the mons, the large lips of the mature female contain fat deposits and hair follicles.

Protected by the large lips are the more delicate *small lips*, although in some cases these protrude past the large lips. The two small lips meet at the top under the mons, and just before they meet they both split into an upper and lower leaf. These embrace the *clitoris*; one leaf passes below the clitoris, the other passes above it, forming a little hood. The clitoris is the anatomical equivalent of the man's penis. It is made up of the same type of erectile tissue which swells with blood during sexual excitement. It is very sensitive to touch, containing many nerve endings, and its sole function is sexual pleasure. Size can vary considerably, although usually it is about the size of a pea. Much of the clitoris is in fact underneath the vulva, so the part of the clitoris that can be felt by your fingers really gives little indication of the actual size of the entire organ.

Beneath the clitoris is the *urethra*, the opening which leads to the bladder.

Below the urethra is the entrance to the *vagina*, which is a muscular tube that stretches upwards and backwards to the *womb* (Figure 2). The vagina passes through a group of muscles which make up the *pelvic floor*. These are a very important muscle group because they support all the contents of the abdomen especially when you stand or exert yourself in any way. The pelvic floor is bounded on each side by the tops of your thighs, and stretches from the tailbone behind to the pubic bone in front.

The first third of the vagina is made up of a strong ring of muscles called the *vaginal sphincter*.

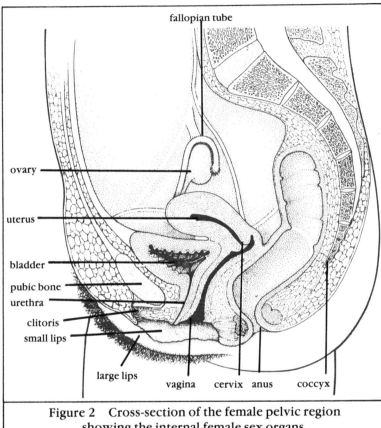

fallopian tube

ovary

uterus

bladder

pubic bone

urethra

clitoris

small lips

large lips

vagina   cervix   anus   coccyx

Figure 2   Cross-section of the female pelvic region
showing the internal female sex organs

This allows the vaginal entrance to remain closed
most of the time, but also to relax and expand when
necessary. The *pubococcygeus* muscle stretches like a
taut hammock from the pubic bone to the coccyx,
looping around the urethra, the anus, and the middle
third of the vagina. As the pubococcygeus muscle is

not a sphincter, the inner portion of the vagina does not have the same grasping action as the vaginal opening. There are other muscle groups which help to make up the vaginal walls, but these are the most important. The various muscles work together to allow the vagina to function effectively during intercourse and childbirth.

The musculature of the vagina is covered by a mucous membrane which contains relatively few nerve endings, so that a woman can run her fingernail down the inside of her vagina and be aware of little sensation.

The primary function of the vagina is as a birth canal. It allows sperm entry to the womb, and the fully developed foetus exit to the outside world. It is also the passage for the discharge of the monthly menstrual flow.

That fact that the womb lies deep within the woman's body is very significant. It means that the developing baby is protected by the powerful muscles which make up the womb, as well as the surrounding musculature and bony structures. The developing young of other species, such as fish, birds and insects are extremely vulnerable as their development takes place outside their mothers' bodies. The human female is a very sophisticated baby-maker!

Protruding from both sides of the top of the womb are the *fallopian tubes*, which extend to lie in contact with the *ovaries*. The ovaries are the equivalent of the male testicles. The ovaries manufacture the female sex hormones oestrogen and progesterone, as well as store the woman's supply of immature eggs (more than 500,000 at birth). Roughly every 28 days, one of those eggs matures and leaves the ovary, making it available for conception. If conception does not occur, around 14 days later the process known as menstruation will begin.

THE MAN

Males tend to know more about their own anatomy compared to women for several good reasons. Their sexual equipment is large, external and in a very obvious position. Also, when a male reaches puberty, his sexual apparatus starts to work of its own accord; the young male has erection and ejaculation without him having to do anything to get the process started. In addition, society generally approves of male sexuality, so he is not as inhibited to learn about himself. Perhaps his main anxiety at this time is whether his penis is large enough — a quite unnecessary worry but one which seems to preoccupy some men who are concerned about their sexual performance.

The male's reproductive role, in contrast to the female's, is quite simple. His sexual apparatus is designed to serve two basic purposes. He has to produce sperm and then deposit it as close as possible to the female's womb, so that conception can occur.

Sperm production takes place in the two *testes*, or testicles (Figure 3). These also make the male sex hormones which cause the bodily changes at puberty. The *epididymis*, attached to the testicle, is where the sperm mature. There is a system of tubes, the *vas*

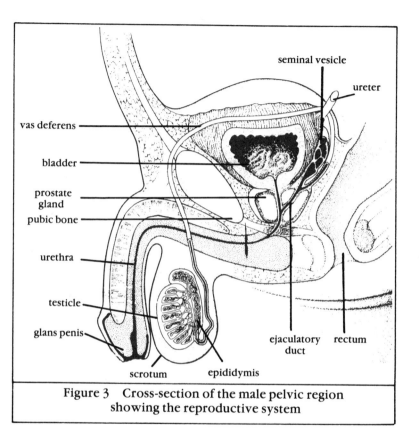

Figure 3   Cross-section of the male pelvic region
showing the reproductive system

deferens, to carry sperm from the testes to the penis. Along these tubes are storage sacs, called *seminal vesicles*. These are necessary because the testes produce sperm continuously, not simply during orgasm. On average, a healthy man will produce about 90 million sperm per day.

Also along the vas deferens are glands which produce the fluid which contains and nourishes the

23

sperm during and after *ejaculation*.

The testes are contained in a wrinkly sac of skin called the *scrotum*. The scrotum is capable of pulling the testes up closer to the body for warmth when it is cold, and lowering the testes in the heat.

The second function of the male sexual organs is to deposit the sperm as close as possible to the female's womb. As was noted earlier, the womb is placed within the female's body for the protection of the growing foetus. But if the sperm were simply deposited on the woman's vulva, few sperm would be strong enough to make the journey up the woman's vagina, through the womb and into the fallopian tubes where conception occurs. So the male has the ability for his penis to become hard enough to be able to penetrate into the woman's vagina. The stimulation of the penis, as it rubs against the walls of the vagina, triggers *ejaculation*, when literally millions of sperm spurt out of the penis towards the neck of the womb.

So it is necessary for the penis to be erect for the process we know as *intercourse* to occur. Erection of the penis is possible because it is made up of columns of spongy tissue which fill with blood during sexual excitement. However, it is also important that the penis is not always erect, for otherwise it would be difficult for the male to urinate. When the male is aroused, a valve shuts off the opening to the bladder so that urine does not escape during orgasm. Most of the time, therefore, the penis is limp and hangs downwards.

WHY DO WE HAVE SEX?

While this may seem like a silly question, it is actually very interesting to try to understand what motivates a man and a woman to cooperate together to perform intercourse.

This motivation to seek sex is called *sex drive* and, despite extensive interest and research, it is not clearly understood. It is interesting to consider some of the facts we do know about this "mysterious" sex drive. Unlike our other drives of hunger and thirst, we do not die if our sex drive is not satisfied. Indeed, it is quite possible for a person to lead a healthy and happy life without any sex drive at all. However, if no-one desired sex and engaged in intercourse, the human race would obviously die out.

Yet we certainly do not have sex merely to produce children, otherwise the contraceptive industry would be out of business.

Do we have sex because our bodies tell us we are sexually frustrated? What does it mean to feel sexually frustrated, or randy? Is this the result of hormones in our bodies?

Certainly, in order to be able to experience sex drive and perform sexual intercourse, certain physical requirements are necessary. These include mature, undamaged genitals, appropriate hormonal development, and intact nerve pathways. If a male, for example, has always had inadequate testosterone levels, he will probably have a very low sex drive and have difficulty becoming aroused. Some diseases, such as diabetes, can seriously affect sexual desire and performance.

Even if the person is physically quite normal, however, he or she may still have a very low sex drive. Sex drive seems to be something we need to learn, rather than simply develop. For example, animals reared in isolation typically do not show normal sexual motivation and behaviour even though they are physically quite normal.

For men and women, too, what they learn about sex, from their family, friends and society, will influence the degree to which they see sex as a worthwhile, enjoyable pursuit. More specifically, we learn to feel randy by practice, which introduces us to the importance of masturbation.

In our society some people think that masturbation is perverted, dirty or in some way abnormal. However, masturbation plays an important role in the development of the sex drive for both men and women. It teaches the maturing person what sexual arousal is and, best of all, how to produce an orgasm.

The pleasurable feeling of orgasm is one of the motivators to encourage a person to seek sex. Without the learning experience provided by masturbation during adolescence, both males and females as adults are likely to have little or no sexual interest.

There is something we need to consider at this point in our discussion. In our society, males typically have a stronger sex drive than women. Is this purely because males and females are taught different things about sex as they are growing up, or is there a biological basis to this difference?

I am prepared to leave myself wide open to criticism by saying that I feel this difference in drive is due to both cultural *and* biological factors.

Certainly in our society males and females learn different things about sex. It is still more acceptable for men to be sexually interested than women. Conversely, it is much easier for a woman to accept the fact that she has a low sex drive than it is for a man.

Teenagers tell me that the old double standard still exists: the male is a "hero" if he admits (or fantasises) frequent sexual experience, whereas the female is still regarded as "slack".

Males read *Penthouse* and *Playboy*, females read Mills and Boon love stories. Men are taught to see the female body as desirable by constant exposure on calendars, advertisements, in movies and in books. But the male body is still hidden. Women do not get the opportunity to see the aroused male body during the years their sex drive should be developing. As a result, they tend not to find the sight of the naked male a powerful trigger for sexual arousal, unlike the male who usually only has to imagine a woman undressing to feel sexually interested.

However, I think there is more to this difference between the sexes than merely the way we are conditioned by society.

To begin with, at puberty males automatically experience sexual arousal, erection and ejaculation which is usually associated with a feeling of pleasure (orgasm). The equivalent biological event for the female is the beginning of ovulation and menstruation. While this may be associated with vague sexual stirrings, it does not have the specific focus experienced by the male and usually goes unrecognised, if it occurs at all. Females do not automatically experience arousal and orgasm. If a male does not discover masturbation, he will at least experience wet dreams. However, females only seem to have orgasmic dreams once they have been sexually active and orgasmic for some considerable time, if at all. Similarly, about 50 per cent of women are aware of feelings of greater sexual interest at certain times during their menstrual cycle. This only seems to develop as the woman becomes more aware of her sexuality, as a result of long-term sexual activity. Therefore, it is extremely difficult to justify the conclusion that the onset of menstruation is associated with an automatic hormonal push to the development of the sex drive, as seems to be the case with males.

Also, the male sexual apparatus is large and obvious. It is very easy for the developing male to discover masturbation which will greatly enhance the development of his sex drive. The female sexual organs are, in contrast, small and hidden, and it is often these factors, rather than embarrassment and inhibition, which stop the female discovering masturbation during her adolescence.

Further, if we look at the male and female roles in the reproduction of the species, the male *must* be aroused in order to perform intercourse. The female, on the other hand, has only to permit intercourse to enable conception to occur. Somewhere along the evolutionary trail it seems to me that the male had to be endowed with a strong physical desire, and to achieve ejaculation and orgasm relatively easily in order to keep the species going. Sexual motivation in the female came to be directed towards permitting intercourse, rather than necessarily seeking it.

Please note, however, that this in no way implies that the female is sexually inferior, only that she is different in some ways. And I am not ignoring research carried out in recent years which has shown that males and females are much more similar than was previously believed. This research suggests that the sexes are more similar than they are different. Nevertheless, this does not rule out the fact that there are some differences between the sexes. It is the lack of appreciation of these differences by both males and females that has caused so many sexual problems for the couple, as we shall see later in the book. Rather than expecting women to be exactly like men, we need to explore what things are likely to encourage a woman to feel like sex. Women are sexual creatures too, but in their own way.

A further biological difference between males and females resides in the fact that males are continuously producing sperm (millions each day) while women ovulate for a brief period once a month. It is not unreasonable to assume that males experience an accumulating physiological pressure which demands release on a fairly regular basis. As the storage sacs along the vas deferens gradually fill, and maximum level is reached, he probably becomes more sensitive to sexual stimuli. If males do not experience sexual release through intercourse or masturbation, they are likely to experience a nocturnal emission (wet dream). However, the influence of practice and learning is evident even here, as it seems that if, over a lengthy period of time, the male decreases his sexual activity of all kinds, then he is also likely to experience a decrease in drive and in nocturnal emissions. This is associated with a decrease in the production of testosterone, the hormone related to strength of sex drive.

So you see the issue is extremely complicated and there is little agreement among experts as to the exact physical basis of the sex drive.

To complicate matters even further, it is also clear that people have sex for a variety of reasons other than just the need for physical release. Even people (males and females) with very strong physical sex drives are not always motivated merely by that. We can decide to have sex for purely emotional reasons, before any physical desire is felt. We might seek sex out of love and caring; the desire to comfort or be comforted, and the need for reassurance; or simply because we are in a good mood.

Similarly, a feeling of physical arousal can easily be squashed by emotions such as fear of failure, feeling foolish, being rejected, or by distraction. And a person with a normally strong sexual desire may well be uninterested in sex if he or she is going through a period of stress such as financial difficulties, or if circumstances mean that sexual expression is inappropriate, as is sometimes the case with an invalided partner.

What we can conclude from all of this is that sex drive is likely to differ greatly from person to person depending on the interaction of all possible contributing factors, both physical and emotional. It seems almost impossible to talk about a "normal" sex drive, although some people seem obsessed with that. Thus, for example, although men seem to have a stronger physical desire for sex than women, it is not, however, unusual to meet women who have developed their sex drive by masturbation, or who simply enjoy expressing themselves physically. Conversely, some men desire sex infrequently, and this need not indicate any problem.

Is it normal to have sex twice a day? Twice a week? Once a month? Only you and your partner can work that one out. I will be dealing with the problem of incompatible sex drives in a later chapter.

WHAT IS SEXUAL AROUSAL AND ORGASM?

Having discussed what motivates a person to have sex, we can now look at what happens to the body during the build-up of arousal and subsequent orgasm.

Before we start, however, I must point out that while a male must be aroused to perform intercourse and usually desires orgasm, this is not always true for the female. We are, therefore, only concerned here with bodily changes when sexual excitement occurs.

It is often assumed that women are slower to become aroused than men. Certainly the experiences of many, in long-term relationships, would seem to bear this out.

However, the famous sex researchers, Masters and Johnson, were able to show that women are capable of reaching orgasm within a few minutes after effective stimulation. The key word here is "effective". Many of the typical foreplay techniques suggested by some sex manuals are not only ineffective, they are downright annoying, as many couples have discovered. Also, because the male seems to have the stronger sex drive, *he* does most of the asking. This means he is already sexually interested when he initiates sex. His partner, on the other hand, may still be planning tomorrow night's menu in her mind and so is somewhat caught out when he starts to make his advances. Naturally, under these circumstances, the woman would lag behind the man in the arousal stakes.

Once both the male and female have begun to be aroused, Masters and Johnson found remarkable similarities between their respective sexual response cycles.

For both sexes, the cycle has four phases: the excitement, plateau, orgasmic and resolution phases.

The *excitement* stage is started by whatever is sexually stimulating for the particular individual. It may be a touch, seeing an available partner, reading something sexy, or merely thinking an erotic thought. If the stimulation is strong enough, excitement builds quickly. If it is interrupted or becomes annoying, this phase becomes extended or the cycle may be stopped. The first physiological response in the male to erotic stimulation is the erection of the penis; in women it is the moistening of the vaginal lining with a lubricating fluid. Other changes in men include further congestion of blood around the scrotum, some elevation of the testes, and increased muscle tension particularly around the genital region. Women experience engorgement of the entire genital region with blood, causing the clitoris to swell, and the beginning of muscle tension in the genital region.

If effective stimulation is continued, it produces increased levels of muscle tension which also becomes more widespread. This increased tension is called the *plateau* phase. If the individual's drive for sexual release in this phase is not strong enough, or if stimulation ceases to be effective or is withdrawn, the person will not experience orgasm. He or she will enter a prolonged period of gradually decreasing sexual tension. This winding-down period in the absence of orgasm may be experienced as a feeling of frustration and discomfort. During the plateau phase, the male testes increase in size by about 50 per cent, and they are pulled up high in the scrotum. For the woman, there is engorgement and swelling of the tissues surrounding the outer third of the vagina; the deeper portion, by contrast, balloons out to form a cavity. The uterus enlarges; the clitoris retracts from its unstimulated position to a relatively inaccessible place under the clitoral hood.

The climactic or *orgasmic* phase, a totally involuntary response, consists of those few seconds when the changes of the body, resulting from stimulation, reach their maximum intensity. The major physical characteristics of orgasm in the female are rhythmic contractions of the outer third of the vagina, and the uterus. The male orgasm is characterised by a series of rhythmic contractions of the urethra, vas and associated tubes and muscles. This is followed by ejaculation of the semen. This occurs in two stages, the first of which is basically the mixing of the various fluids which contribute to the ejaculation, and the second is the actual expulsion of the ejaculate from the penis. In both males and females, various muscle groups throughout the body may also contract during orgasm.

During the *resolution* phase, after orgasm, there is a lessening of sexual tension as the person returns to the unstimulated state. Women are capable of having another orgasm if there is effective stimulation during this phase. The resolution phase in the male includes a time, which varies among individuals, when re-stimulation is impossible. This is called the refractory period.

MORE ABOUT ORGASM

In the last section we talked about the physical side of arousal and orgasm. What does orgasm feel like?

As every other author who has written on the subject has said, it is almost impossible to adequately describe what orgasm feels like to different individuals. But I do not agree with these other authors when they say that if a woman is unsure whether or not she has had an orgasm, then she probably hasn't.

This is because they are thinking only about the top-of-the-range type orgasm, which is quite unmistakable. This is the orgasm that novelists describe in detailed delight and actors and actresses portray with enthusiasm.

But there are varieties of orgasm. Many orgasms are very run-of-the-mill, nowhere near the top of the range, some so low key that the woman is not necessarily aware that it has happened except that she feels somewhat sleepy and relaxed. One woman told me she had never had an orgasm but she did often have a nice "trembly" feeling during foreplay. She was most surprised to find that she was experiencing orgasm. "But," she said, "it's nothing like you see in the movies."

Males do not have the same problem of deciding whether they reach orgasm or not, since they actually ejaculate "proof" of their response. However, men are often aware of enjoying ejaculation more or less depending on their mood and can notice that there is sometimes little or no pleasure associated with ejaculation. Orgasm for the male is the pleasure associated with the physical process of ejaculation. When men think of their own experience in this way, it can help them to be aware of the varying strengths of orgasm that women experience.

Although there are undoubtedly times when a woman unknowingly experiences a "mini-orgasm", nevertheless, it is true that few women reach orgasm during every sexual encounter. There is some disagreement in the research literature as to just how many women can achieve orgasm by what means, and how often. However, it is clear that there are many women who experience orgasm on only an irregular basis, and some who do not come to orgasm at all.

There are two points to be considered here. The first is that women need to learn to orgasm. The inappropriate sexual training females receive in our culture is the single most important contributor to the orgasmic difficulties experienced by probably the majority of women in Australia at the present time. I am confident that with appropriate sex education, most young girls would develop the ability to orgasm without too much difficulty.

The second point to consider is that there is agreement from many studies that women do not need to come to orgasm to enjoy intercourse. This emphasis on the orgasmic response is creating a very rigid stereotype of female sexuality. Unlike males, women do not need to be aroused to perform intercourse. From an evolutionary point of view, the male orgasm was essential, the female orgasm largely irrelevant. This has created the situation where it seems more difficult for women to develop the orgasmic response compare to men. Nevertheless, I think it is extremely pessimistic thinking to see this as a flaw in female sexuality. What it means is that a female's response to a sexual situation is more flexible by virtue of the very fact that she does not need to be aroused. She has a whole range of options, from the low-key possibility of using artificial lubrication as an aid to gentle, passive lovemaking, to the highly aroused state where she is the initiator and most active participant. The male, by contrast, would find it very difficult to easily substitute an artificial erection.

Some men have pointed out to me that men can also enjoy love-play without arousal and orgasm, and this may well be true. Nevertheless, in perhaps female chauvinistic fashion, I suspect that this is more the exception than the rule, whereas for women it is an *integral* part of their sexuality.

One of Masters and Johnson's findings underscores this point. They found that under conditions of fatigue or anxiety, the time taken for the female to reach orgasm *increases*; for the male, assuming he is able to obtain an erection, time taken to orgasm tends to *decrease*. When a woman is feeling even slightly negative, it becomes more difficult for her to come to orgasm. So why should she bother, when it can be more pleasurable to focus on the other apparently forgotten aspects of a sexual encounter, such as a feeling of calmness and intimacy.

Another interesting question to examine is how a woman achieves orgasm, and whether she ejaculates when she does so. With males there is no disagreement as to the nature of arousal, ejaculation and orgasm. With women, there is continual debate as to whether all orgasms are the same, whether they are achieved by direct stimulation of the clitoris versus penile thrusting in the vagina, or whether different mechanisms are involved depending on the type of stimulation. Current surveys suggest that in our society most women do not achieve orgasm with penile thrusting. Rather, arousal and orgasm is more reliably achieved by direct clitoral stimulation during foreplay. Masters and Johnson claimed that even during intercourse the clitoris was indirectly stimulated by tension on the small lips as a result of penile penetration and thrusting, and it was this stimulation that ultimately led to orgasm.

However, other sex researchers feel that an orgasm achieved through penile thrusting occurs by a different means. Certainly, women who can come to orgasm by both methods report that the orgasms *feel* different, so perhaps they do have a different physical basis. The proponents of the vaginal orgasm fall into two camps. The first has been around the longest, even before Masters and Johnson. In the early 1950s a doctor called Kegel developed a set of exercises for the muscles of the pelvic floor (basically, the musculature of the vulval-anal region). He originally intended these exercises to be used for women with urinary incontinence, but he discovered a curious side effect. Many of his patients reported that after several months of regular exercise, they began to experience much more response during inter-course. Earlier in this chapter I mentioned that the mucous membrane lining the vagina has few nerve endings and is therefore quite insensitive. However, the muscles underneath the membrane have a plentiful supply of nerve endings. Hence the argument is that by toning up the muscles around the vagina, they offer more resistance during penile thrusting, thus stimulating the nerve endings by this pressure. This school of thought argues that only by having good tone in the muscles of the pelvic floor is vaginal orgasm possible.

The second school of thought on the concept of vaginal orgasm has gained favour much more re-cently. It is tied up with the notion of female eja-culation. Since 1978, a number of research papers have been published claiming that some women actually *do* ejaculate a fluid during orgasm. These researchers claim that some women appear to have a gland that could best be described as a primitive prostate, and that during orgasm it squirts fluid into the urethra, which expels it onto the vulval area. The area in which this gland can be located is known as the Grafenberg spot, after a German gynaecologist who, in the 1950s, described an especially sensitive area inside the vagina. This "spot" is located in the front wall of the vagina and can only be stimulated by strong pressure, such as could be achieved by intercourse in the rear entry position. According to the researchers, pressure on the Grafenberg spot produces an intense orgasmic response in the woman, apparently without the need for extended foreplay.

This research is new and has yet to be widely accepted. However, if a woman feels comfortable allowing her partner to explore her vagina with his fingers (which is apparently the only way to initially locate the spot) and does find that pressure in a particular spot produces orgasm and a type of ejaculation, then this would seem to be an added bonus to female sexuality.

It is obvious that there is still a lot we do not know about orgasm in particular and sexuality in general. For this reason, no book should be regarded as the final word on sex. I hope this chapter has developed your curiosity about your body and how it works, so that you will keep reading new works long after this one has disappeared from the shelves.

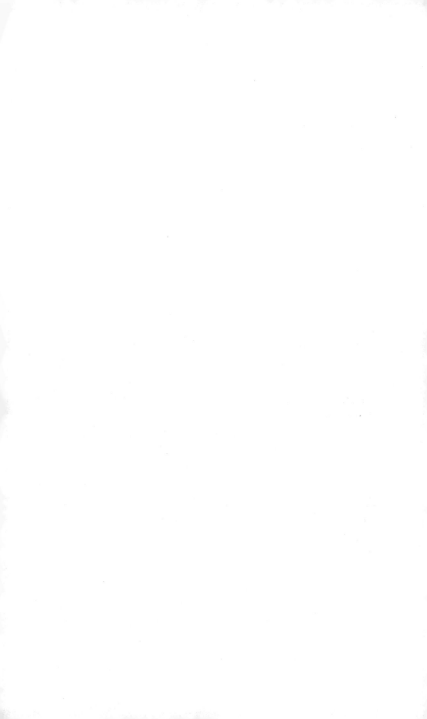

1. A couple should have sex frequently, at least a couple of times a week, and preferably every night.

This belief ignores the fact that we cannot separate sexual desire from the daily crisis of a sick child, or problems at work, or financial difficulties. During these times it is quite normal to be less interested in sex. But even normal fluctuations in tiredness, for example, from spending the day working in the garden, will influence your desire for sex. This is particularly true for women.

Therefore, it is not unreasonable or unusual for a couple to go several days or even weeks without intercourse. Usually frequency fluctuates, perhaps occurring three times one week and not at all the next.

For some couples, a frequency of once or twice a month can be quite satisfying and should not be regarded as abnormal. Problems arise when each partner has different sexual drives, and this will be discussed in Chapter 4.

2. Both partners should enjoy sexual stimulation, arouse easily, and come to orgasm often.

We saw in Chapter 2 that when a woman is tired, her time to orgasm increases, while a male's decreases. In fact it becomes hard work for a woman to turn on if she is feeling at all negative. She is then quite likely to find any form of sexual stimulation (breast or genital) quite annoying, in contrast to the male who usually finds it quite soothing. What this means is that sexual stimulation aimed at arousal is often inappropriate for the female. The couple might do better if they concentrated on relaxing and comforting caresses instead. Women do not need to come to orgasm to enjoy sex.

The male, too, often enjoys relaxing and comforting foreplay and does not always require direct sexual stimulation to become aroused. So gentle, reassuring lovemaking is quite possible.

3. Exciting sex is best.

This particular myth gives us an extremely limited view of the pleasure of sex.

In the pursuit of physical excitement, the other pleasures of sex have been overlooked. I mentioned gentle, reassuring lovemaking in the last section. Sometimes it is truly delightful to *make love* to the other person rather than being concerned about arousal and orgasm. By this I mean the expression of affection and caring, to touch and talk to this person like a treasured friend rather than to regard him/her as merely a means to an orgasm. Often the emphasis on physical arousal gets in the way of this emotional intercourse, yet in a long-term relationship the emotional contact is at least equally as important.

The other point to consider is that if we believe that only exciting sex is acceptable, two things happen. Firstly, we avoid sex unless we are sure we can turn on, so we miss all those opportunities for peaceful, relaxing lovemaking. Secondly, sex becomes hard work — which in my opinion is a complete waste of time. It is nice to know that sex is sometimes delightfully, blessedly dull, that it is OK not to try hard all the time. Even falling asleep during sex sometimes can be a nice sexual response. This is obviously easier for the woman to do, but even the

although their sexuality is an integral part of their self-image. Women, on the other hand, have traditionally been allowed to be emotional but have been repressed sexually. This leads to a "crossed-wires" situation. Men find it easier to express themselves sexually rather than emotionally, whereas for women it is typically the other way around.

Thus it seems that males often use sex as a means of expressing emotion. They are usually not, as many women fear, simply wanting to have sex for sexual release. So, if he has the greater sex drive, he seeks sex more often than the woman wants. This makes her feel sexually inadequate by comparison, but at the same time when she turns him down he feels rejected emotionally. What a mess!

We can clear this up quite simply by recognising a few simple facts. Firstly, at the present time the male is more likely to want sex more often than the female (hopefully we can change this with proper sex education). This means that he is going to seek sex at least on some occasions when his partner does not feel like it at all, so it is reasonable that she will want to say no. If you think about it, both do not always feel happy at the same moment, or depressed, or irritated, so it stands to reason that both are not always going to feel sexy at the same time. Therefore, to say no to sex is merely expressing a statement of fact, that she (or he) does not feel sexy. It has nothing to do with personal rejection. Obviously the same applies if it is the woman who has the higher drive.

We also have to consider when and how the sexual approach is made. Unfortunately, this is usually last thing at night when the other partner is very likely to be tired and the approach is very often direct ("How about it?", or a touch of the breast) which only produces a groan of annoyance. So saying no under these conditions should come as no surprise.

The final point to consider here is how the "no" is said. If it is: "For heaven's sake leave me alone", it is no wonder the other partner feels rejected. But an "I don't feel sexy, but I'd love a cuddle" will go a long way to making your partner feel wanted.

7. Men should know what turns a woman on; communicating about likes and dislikes is unnecessary and insulting.

This idea comes across so often in many movie scenes. The man is usually the initiator, and without any dialogue the film rolls on to suggest hours of endless pleasure, with every movement made by the man producing exquisite delight for the female.

It is often also related to the belief that "if he loved me he would know".

But it is impossible for a sexual relationship to survive without clear communication. This does not mean that you and your partner must have a half-hour planning session before every sexual encounter. It does mean that you can say "that's nice", or "not there, here", or move a hand to where you want it, without it meaning that your partner is inadequate for not automatically knowing.

Sexual needs and desires can change from day to day, particularly for the female, who seems to be more influenced by mood. How can your partner know what you need or enjoy without telling him

WHAT, THEN, IS A GOOD SEXUAL RELATIONSHIP?

To start with, I define a good sexual relationship not so much in terms of what the couple are doing when things are going well, but how they cope together when things are not so good.

A sexual relationship in which both partners always feel like sex, and both can arouse and come to orgasm when they want, is certainly to be admired. And I suppose there are sex gourmets who devote their time and energy to achieving an exciting and varied sex life, in much the same way that food gourmets and wine buffs relentlessly pursue their particular obsessions.

However, few people lead charmed lives, or are in a position to place their sexual needs above all other considerations. Routine problems and unexpected crises must arise from time to time with the majority of couples. Is their sexual relationship, then, a refuge together from the stress, or does it become a barrier between them?

A good sexual relationship does not mean that the couple must always be super-lovers. Rather, a good sexual relationship is flexible enough to adjust to the changing pattern of desires and needs. To my mind, the hallmark of a good sexual relationship is the ability of the couple to compromise and to adjust their expectations to realistic levels so that their sex lives are as hassle-free as possible. For example, one partner may totally withdraw from "arousing sex" for a long period of time, needing passive sex for comfort and reassurance. Is their relationship strong enough to cope with this?

Do they feel comfortable with saying no to sex occasionally, snuggling together to go to sleep instead? Can they solve a disagreement between them (for example, one wants to try a new technique) without it always ending in an almighty row? Is each partner comfortable with his/her own sexuality, and does not feel compelled to prove anything? Does each partner care about the enjoyment of the other, and be willing to change or compromise where appropriate? Do they listen to each other?

All these things are far more important than whether she can orgasm during intercourse, or he can delay ejaculation indefinitely.

This is not to deny that there are specific sexual problems, only, hopefully, to put them in perspective.

Obviously, if your partner is always saying no, or the woman is always aroused but misses orgasm, or the man cannot usually get an erection, or your partner always lies rigid and passive during intercourse, it is realistic that this will put a strain on your relationship at both the sexual and emotional levels. Hopefully, before the problems become too destructive, you and your partner will decide to do something about them. Start with the information in this book, but if you do not get anywhere do not hesitate to seek help from a qualified counsellor or therapist.

Perhaps surprisingly, many couples I have seen over the years with quite severe sexual problems have ultimately developed a very strong, supportive emotional relationship and a satisfying sexual re-

home. Brian came to see me because he had begun masturbating during the week, usually while he was still in bed in the morning and Sue was at work. He had not masturbated in the 15 years since their marriage, and he believed that his masturbation meant that he was becoming sexually perverted. He had not connected the sudden drop in sexual frequency with his urge to masturbate, and did not realise that masturbation was a healthy and normal outlet for sexual frustration.

Paul and Lesley were a couple who had thought they had a good sex life until they read a magazine article that made them feel they must have a problem. They simply were not interested in all the techniques and positions described, and often went for a fortnight or more without sex. This couple needed to disregard what they had read and have enough confidence in themselves to decide what they wanted from their sexual relationship.

So, before you assume that you have a complex, serious sexual problem, sit down and think, logically. What is happening in your life? Do you have a lifestyle problem instead of a sexual problem?

TYPES OF SEXUAL PROBLEM

Once you have decided that there is a sexual problem which is not merely a reflection of lifestyle, or unrealistic ideas about sex, it is then necessary to find out exactly what the problem is. Then a decision can be made as to what to do about it.

To do this, it is helpful to divide sexual functioning into four categories: drive, performance, orgasm and enjoyment.

By *drive*, I mean how interested is the person in having sex? If it was left up to him or her, how often would that person seek intercourse? As I have pointed out already, women seem to have more difficulties with drive than men. I think this is a reflection of biological differences and cultural conditioning, as discussed in Chapter 2. For some women, lack of drive is their only problem, and once sex is initiated, they respond well. For others it is only part of the difficulty. Despite it being mainly a female problem, however, men, too, can have difficulty with drive.

Performance problems refer to difficulties in actually having intercourse, and male sexual problems more commonly fall into this category. Probably the most common male sexual problem is premature ejaculation, which means that the male ejaculates prior to or immediately after penetration of the vagina. The other major male problem is impotence, which means that he has difficulty achieving or maintaining an erection.

Performance problems for women are either painful intercourse, or the inability to have intercourse at all. This latter condition is known as vaginismus, and means the woman is unable to relax her vagina sufficiently to permit intercourse to take place.

Difficulties with *orgasm* are predominantly a female problem, although there are males who, despite being aroused, do not enjoy ejaculation. Some women have never achieved orgasm, and some only achieve orgasm in specific situations such as with self-stimulation, or during foreplay.

Problems with *enjoyment* of sex may simply be the result of problems in other areas, and once these problems are solved, enjoyment increases. Or, lack of enjoyment may indicate communication problems, or difficulties in the caring relationship. Lack of enjoyment can be a problem even though both partners achieve orgasm easily.

These, then, are the broad categories to look at when trying to break your sexual problem down into manageable units. In the following chapters I will deal with each of these categories in detail so that you can begin to work your way out of your problem.

Before treatment for any of these sexual problems is considered, you need to realise that best results are achieved if both partners are concerned enough to cooperate to solve the difficulty. Although one partner may be the person with the obvious difficulty, it is usually a joint problem. So talk about it with your partner. Having a sexual problem is not such a big deal, so there is no need to feel embarrassed or inadequate. Cooperating to solve your problems can actually strengthen your relationship, even though it may be difficult at first. And besides, many of your friends, relatives and neighbours are having similar problems, so you need not feel abnormal.

If you and your partner do try to solve your sexual problems, be prepared for some misunderstandings and disagreements. *But remember, it is impossible to argue someone out of a sexual problem.*

However, people can often change with caring support and encouragement.

So give it a go. I am not expecting you to do anything that you do not want to, or that you feel is wrong. It is up to you and your partner to decide what is appropriate for you as a couple. The aim of this book is for you to gain enough self-confidence by acquiring appropriate information, to develop the type of sex life that suits you and your partner.

4 PROBLEMS WITH DRIVE

When a couple feels that one or both of them has a problem with sex drive, they should not automatically assume that the person with the lower drive has a major sexual problem.

We need to know a lot more about the how, when, where and why of the situation before jumping to any conclusions.

For example, it is important to know whether the person, male or female, *ever* wants sex, and if so, under what circumstances. Sometimes it may be the partner who is demanding sex too often that is the cause of the problem. It is important to remember that the cultural expectation that a person should feel like sex every night or every second night is often unrealistic.

On the other hand, both partners may have healthy, reasonable sex drives, but unfortunately they do not match up very well. And remember, it does not matter how often or how rarely a couple have sex. If you and your partner are having sex at a frequency that suits you both, whether it is twice a day or twice a year, then you do not have a problem.

FEMALE LACK OF DRIVE

Probably the most common of all sexual problems

among women is low or absent sex drive. Many women describe their problem by saying: "If it wasn't for my husband, I wouldn't care if I never had sex again." Each is convinced that she is frigid, and that it must be the result of some major trauma somewhere in her history.

It is certainly possible that for some women, by far in the minority, their sexual problem is the result of a trauma in their past. In my experience, however, these women do not present with a single symptom such as disinterest in sex. They often find all aspects of sex unpleasant, sometimes bringing on feelings of panic, disgust or revulsion. These women will probably not find this book very useful, and I would encourage each of them to discuss her problems with a qualified health professional. Remember, even these more serious problems have developed for a good reason, so do not be afraid or embarrassed to seek help.

On the other hand, simply not feeling like sex, or being irritated or annoyed by attempts at arousal, are not good enough reasons to assume that you have a serious psychological problem. These symptoms are so common amongst women in our society that they are usually indicators of a healthy woman brought up in a society where inhibition and sensationalism muddy our understanding of sexuality in general, and female sexuality in particular.

Therefore, take heart. Let's try to work out what is happening with you, and see what can be done about it. To do this, I'll ask a series of questions, just as I would if I were seeing you in my office. By reading the explanations and suggestions given to the possible replies, you and your partner will be able to develop ideas on how to start helping yourself.

GROUP I QUESTIONS
1. *Do you ever feel like sex?*
2. *Did you at any time in the past feel more like sex than you do now?*
3. *Can you remember masturbating during adolescence?*
4. *What were your parents' attitudes to sex as you were growing up?*
5. *Can you come to orgasm now, by any means at all?*
6. *Can you orgasm easily, or is it a lot of hard work?*
7. *Do you usually enjoy sex once you get started, or is it usually unenjoyable throughout?*

This group of questions helps to describe your problem more accurately and so give a clearer picture of some possible factors in your low sex drive. There are a number of possible characteristics to any particular woman's problem, depending on her answers to these and other questions. Nevertheless, there are a number of common pictures which emerge to account for most cases of low sex drive in women.

Type A: The first type we will consider is the woman who has *never* felt like sex in the past, and certainly can't be bothered with it now. The best she hopes for is that her partner does not approach her too often and when he does he gets it over and done with quickly. This woman typically did not masturbate during adolescence, and cannot come to orgasm by any means now. As a growing teenager she was not necessarily told anything bad about sex, but she certainly was not told anything good. She tended to believe that premarital sex was not right, although she may have gone along with her partner to please him.

She simply cannot understand why on earth her partner wants sex as often as he does, and she sometimes feels hurt because she thinks he might only be using her for sexual release.

The problem with this woman is that she was brought up in a sexual vacuum. We know that to develop into healthy mature sexual adults, sexual learning should occur naturally throughout life. Certainly during adolescence, sexual curiosity is normal and healthy. The growing adolescent should be encouraged to read straightforward (*not* sensational) sex education books, be able to discuss sexual matters openly with her parents, and ideally feel comfortable with masturbation. This woman has missed out on all of this, so it is no wonder she finds sex an annoying thing to do.

Type B: This woman is similar to Type A, except that at one time in her life she did feel like sex more often than she does now.

Not uncommonly, it might have been before she and her partner were living together. Then, she was living at home with Mum and Dad. All she had to worry about was going to work, and going out socially. Mum took care of all the housework. When she was going out with her boyfriend, she would come home from work, eat dinner, then shower and get dressed. He would pick her up and they would spent an enjoyable evening together, appreciating their special relationship. Later on, he would initiate petting and intercourse, and she would enjoy it (although possibly not climax) because she was feeling relaxed and emotionally close to her partner.

Compare this to the postmarriage scene. Both are working full-time, money is tight as they try to save for a house, she has to prepare dinner when she gets home from work, and then tidy up afterwards. After dinner she catches up on the washing and cleaning, and maybe he gives her a hand or else has to go to technical college, university, or out to squash. They sit watching television most nights without saying more than a dozen words, then they fall into bed and expect to feel like sex. Every now and again she finds sex OK, and even, perhaps, on rare occasions, can come to orgasm, but this is usually quite difficult.

Other common life events which can have a detrimental effect on the woman's sexual desire can be the birth of a child, financial problems, prolonged sickness either of herself or a family member, and so on. All these events usually make the woman feel more tired, or worried, or hassled, and will often cause a drop in sexual desire.

The problem here is that during adolescence, her sex drive was never very strong for similar reasons as woman A. Therefore, it does not take very much to push it down again. But even very robust sex drives will suffer if the life event has a marked impact on the woman's well-being.

Type C: This is the final type we will consider, although you might find you do not fit any of the three types exactly. The individual variations are too numerous to describe in detail.

Woman C had quite a reasonable sex drive at one time, and often masturbated during adolescence. She could come to orgasm with masturbation, but, nevertheless, worried whether she was perverted for doing it. As a result of her adolescent behaviour, woman C can come to orgasm easily now with self-stimulation, and also during foreplay with her partner, although this might take a bit of effort. Her problem is only that she never actually feels like sex. Once she actually decides to have sex, she usually starts to become aroused and, even if she does not orgasm, almost always enjoys herself.

This woman tends to confuse her partner greatly. She never approaches him for sex, and is often irritated when he tries to initiate it. Yet, sometimes when he persists despite her initial protests, she becomes quite aroused and thoroughly enjoys herself. Other times, however, she becomes increasingly annoyed, and they can end up in an argument. He never knows what to do to please her, and becomes upset because she won't, or can't, tell him. Some partners react by feeling hurt and rejected, and ultimately avoiding attempts to initiate sex. Others become blasé about the woman's initial irritation and keep trying to get her interested regardless of what she says or does, which only adds to her desire to avoid sexual contact.

As with woman B, over the years something has changed to suppress woman C's sex drive, or the right things aren't being done to get her interested. This brings us to the role played by her partner.

GROUP II QUESTIONS

Before we begin, we need to have one point understood. This part is not an "aren't all men terrible, look what they are doing to their poor women" segment. The purpose of these questions is only to gain a greater understanding of what is happening between you and your partner, not to dish out blame.

Although there are certainly some mean, selfish men, just as there are some inconsiderate women, most men I see are concerned, caring people who simply cannot understand why their female partners don't want sex. After all, *they* do, without any effort at all. In the end, in the absence of sensible information and down-to-earth advice, she believes he is a sex maniac and he thinks she is frigid. We must remember that men have no better sex education than women, and that he is subjected to far more cultural pressure than a woman to be sexually "successful". Often he feels totally confused, and in his confusion and emotional frustration he can become withdrawn and at times aggressive. Yet most men welcome the chance to sort out the problems in their sexual relationship.

1. *Who usually initiates sex? How? When? Where?*
2. *Do you and/or your partner believe that you should always try to be aroused during sex?*
3. *Do you and your partner usually communicate to each other what you like and do not like during foreplay?*

4. *Do you ever say no to your partner's sexual advances, and if so, what happens when you do?*
5. *How often do you think other couples have sex? How often does your partner?*
6. *Do you often stop yourself cuddling your partner because you think he will take this as a sign to try for sex?*
7. *Do you and your partner spend much time alone together, relaxing, talking, cuddling, without it leading to sex?*
8. *Do you worry that your partner just uses you for his sexual satisfaction, not caring about how you feel?*
9. *Do you and/or your partner think you are "frigid"?*
10. *Does he try to understand your point of view and try to help?*
11. *Does your partner have any annoying personal habits that turn you off?*

From this group of questions, you can gain some understanding of the way you and your partner interact, which can be contributing to the problem.

Typically it is the man who does all the asking. Usually, the approach is made in bed at night (after all, the kids are always around at other times or there is something good on television). Often the first the woman knows of his intentions is when he says; "How about it?", or something similar, or else puts his hand on her breast. Often the man tries hard to get his partner interested and aroused, believing that he has let her down in some way if he doesn't.

This couple do not communicate well during lovemaking. He might ask her what she would like, but all she can tell him is what she doesn't like. The woman often says no to her partner's advances, and this typically makes him feel hurt and rejected, and her guilty.

They both tend to think that other couples have sex much more often than they do, but one important thing that puts more strain on their relationship is that they do not cuddle very much. The woman often avoids any attempts at cuddles or a kiss from her partner because he seems to get aroused so easily and she thinks he will want to go on to sex. Because of this, their relationship may not be very close, and they do not spend much time together relaxing or chatting.

Sometimes in their confusion about their sexual relationship, she thinks he tries to have sex with her to ease his sexual frustration. Perhaps by now he believes she has a problem, but he often does try to help. The trouble is, the things he does to help often aggravate the situation.

Occasionally, another part of the woman's reluctance to have sex is due to a personal habit of her partner that turns her off. An unshaven face, an unwashed body, a beery breath, are all common things which women complain about. Sometimes the man is unaware of his partner's feelings, sometimes she nags him to the point where he refuses to budge. But if you want your sex life to improve, you are going to have to find some way of discussing it calmly and getting something done.

This is a composite picture of many sexual relationships where the woman doesn't feel like sex. Your relationship may be quite different in some of the details, but chances are at least some of this description fits the way you and your partner are relating at the moment.

GROUP III QUESTIONS

1. *What, if anything, makes you more likely to feel like sex?*
2. *Does your mind wander during sex?*
3. *Can you fantasise about sexual things?*
4. *How do you feel about planning sex, for example, when you know the kids are going to be away for the night?*
5. *What happens if you are enjoying foreplay but then you are interrupted, say, by the telephone?*
6. *Is there anything happening in your life at the moment that is worrying you, or affects your feelings of well-being?*
7. *Why do you want to change?*

While these questions may seem unrelated, often one or more of them is significant to an individual woman's problem.

The problem with some women is that they have never given a lot of thought to what makes them feel more like sex. She usually says she does not know, but on further probing she realises that having her hair combed, or her back tickled, or whatever, does make her feel more receptive sometimes. Because these are not the sort of things mentioned in sex books, she lacks the confidence to tell her partner how she feels.

Often, a woman with low drive has sex when she really is not interested, or has not had relaxation foreplay, and finds that her mind wanders onto all sorts of irrelevant topics. She might start planning tomorrow night's menu, or suddenly remember that the garbage has not been taken out, and this is somewhat disconcerting to her partner! She usually cannot have sexual fantasies, unlike her partner who seems to her to be able to have them at almost any time of the day.

She usually resents planning sex, partly because she believes sex should be spontaneous, but mainly because she is reluctant to commit herself to something she is quite sure she is not going to feel like anyway. So while the man smiles in anticipation at the thought of the children going to Grandma's for the weekend, she starts to feel tense and annoyed before they have even left. For the same reason, a relaxing evening such as going to dinner often does not produce the desired result because she has spent all three courses feeling agitated by the knowledge that her partner is hoping that when they get home, surely she will feel like it tonight.

If she is having sex and starting to feel a little involved, an interruption spells disaster. A male often seems to have the remarkable ability to put himself on "hold", so that after a 15-minute telephone conversation he will come back and say: "Now, where were we?" By this time she has switched off completely and the chances of rekindling any interest are very likely going to be close to zero.

I have mentioned before that what is happening in your life affects your sexuality, so you need to think calmly about what does get you down, and thus might be affecting your general feeling of well-being. While such life stresses as living with your parents may not be the original cause of the problem, they may mean that things are not going to improve much in the near future.

Finally, you need to think about why you want to tackle the problem of your lack of interest in sex. If it is merely for your partner's sake, think again. It will be easier to change if you want to for *your* sake. It feels nice to want sex, to feel randy sometimes. And, although good sex does not necessarily make a good relationship, bad sex is often the thin end of the wedge between the couple. To enjoy touching and being touched by someone you care about makes life that much more enjoyable.

Right, then, what do you do about all this?

So far, I have merely described the common elements of most cases of low or absent sexual desire in women. Hopefully, I have made you aware that there is more to this problem than just saying, "I'm frigid". There are many factors which may all be important to your understanding of why you cannot be bothered with sex; undoubtedly I have left some out.

Sometimes these factors are simple things, not at all deep and mysterious. Forget what you have seen on the soapies, think simply and you may come up with some surprising answers. One woman, for example, realised that the single most important factor was that she hated being cold, but they usually made love naked and uncovered. Solution: warm the room first. Another woman had enjoyed premarital sex, but after a few months of marriage it had begun to lose its appeal. Finally, after some trial and error, she realised that premaritally she had always made love naked, postmaritally her husband simply pulled her nightie up. She felt very constricted and uncomfortable!

Usually, however, the problem is not quite so straightforward. Before you start tackling your problem, you and your partner need to be aware of, and discuss, one very important fact. There is no magic solution to most sexual problems. Despite what you may have read, instant cures like hypnosis and hormone therapy are usually not the answer. You and your partner need to cooperate so that your sexual relationship will gradually improve over time.

When you think about it, this makes sense. Here you are, an adult, just starting to learn what you should have been developing naturally throughout your life. If it takes 15 to 20 years for a girl to mature under the right circumstances into a sexually responsive adult, you can hardly expect yourself to change overnight. In my experience, it can take several months, sometimes a couple of years, before you find that sexual desire comes easily and often. But, cheer up, there is more to your sexual relationship than that, so in the meantime you and your partner can still be enjoying yourselves if you start using a bit of commonsense.

To begin to improve your sexual relationship, we must start with the basic assumption that men and women are different. It does not matter whether this is a biological or cultural phenomenon, the sexes generally do differ in some areas of sexuality.

One of the most important differences, one that generates tremendous chaos in many sexual relationships, is this:

Women need to feel good before they can respond sexually, whereas men often seek sex in order to feel good.

Read this again, several times. Think about it. What does it mean? I'll give you some common examples.

Example 1: The woman is washing the dishes. Her partner comes up behind her, starts to cuddle and caress her, and wants her to give him a kiss. How would you feel about this? Many women I talk to tell me they feel like decking him with the dish mop.

Compare this with:

He, the man, is fixing the car. He is staring into the engine when the woman comes up behind him and slips her hands down the front of his trousers. He seems much more likely to say, "Hmm, that's nice", even if he is not interested in doing anything about it.

Example 2: The woman is asked by her partner, "How about it? Want to make love?" She replies, perhaps slightly irritated: "Now? Hmm, well, I don't know. Maybe."

He is asked the same question. His reply is likely to be a straightforward "Yes", but if he does not feel like it, or it is not convenient he is likely to say, "No, but how about later?"

Example 3: Early in the evening, the couple has had an argument that has not really been settled. In bed that night, he makes sexual advances. She says:

"But we have just had an argument, how can you expect me to make love to you?" He says: "What has that got to do with it?"

These examples are obviously generalisations. Nevertheless, they seem to ring true for many couples. Probably the greatest impact this difference between the sexes has on a couple's sexual relationship relates to the how, when, where and why that sex is initiated.

The "how"

Unfortunately, for the vast majority of couples in our society, what they have read in various magazines and books about ways of initiating sex and techniques of foreplay is entirely inappropriate for many women.

The culturally accepted idea of the best way to initiate sex revolves around direct sexual stimulation. For many males this means touching the woman's breasts or genitals. It is not unreasonable for them to think this way, because they themselves usually like to be touched around the genital area. However, so many women complain that they find this annoying, irritating or unpleasant, unless they are in the mood for sex, that we have to rethink our ideas.

I can almost guarantee that if she is sitting on the lounge, thinking about all the things she has to do tomorrow, and he sits beside her and starts fondling her breasts, she is going to be somewhat put out about this. On the other hand, if, for example, she has been reading a sexy book and is feeling somewhat interested, then she is much more likely to enjoy this type of stimulation.

Unfortunately, many women never, or only rarely, feel randy because of something they have read, seen or are thinking. Part of the problem here is that, due to lack of masturbation and encouragement to think sexually during adolescence, women in our society have some difficulty thinking erotically. So, they tend not to have sexual fantasies while they are sweeping the floor or preparing dinner. Men, on the other hand, apparently find it much easier to conjure up sexual images, partly because of practice during masturbation, so for this reason they tend to be thinking of sexual things more often. They also get more cues of sexual frustration from their bodies.

So, he feels randy, and sex seems like a good idea, particularly with this woman he cares about. The idea of touching her breasts or putting his hand down her pants is very appealing.

But for the woman, particularly one with low drive, the most important foreplay she needs are things that make her feel relaxed, to give her a chance to switch off from the day's events. This might mean being left alone for a while after getting the children to bed, or having a shower (alone), or having a cup of coffee together, having her shoulders rubbed, chatting with her partner. Anything that she enjoys that makes her feel relaxed and helps her think nice thoughts about the person she is with, is appropriate.

Without this, attempts at arousal are either very difficult, or a waste of time.

What I am asking you both to do is to completely rethink your ideas about what is likely to make the woman feel that sex isn't such a bad idea after all. For the woman with low drive, in the early stages of working on your problem, there is no point in trying anything else in foreplay but these relaxing things.

For the man, try to appreciate that she will want to have sex more often if you initiate it the way *she* likes, not the way the books say she *should* like. But this means being able to communicate positively, and without fear of hurting or insulting each other. You cannot know what she feels like unless she tells you, so she needs to give you some clues as to what does feel nice on this occasion.

This is very important when we realise that women often vary tremendously from night to night. One night she really responds to, for example, breast stimulation; the next night it only produces a groan of annoyance. Some nights she is initially irritated but then becomes aroused, other nights the longer he tries to arouse her the more annoyed she becomes. Clear communication is the only key to solve this problem. Even then it is still difficult to overcome the confusion when she is initially adamant that she is *not* interested but then turns on when he persists. So, the couple have to be realistic and not let the occasional conflict affect other attempts to initiate sex. She needs to keep trying to develop confidence to be able to tell him on every occasion what she feels like, and he needs to be confident enough to listen and respond.

The "when"

At the present time, the average couple (particularly those with children) typically have sex late in the evening. I can understand why this seems the best time, but in fact it is the worst time for sexual arousal. If the man is very tired he might have some difficulty achieving an erection, if he is a little tired he will tend to ejaculate rapidly. Nevertheless, he is still likely to think that sex (and for him, that also means orgasm) is the best sedative around. From the woman's point of view, arousal is very difficult when she is tired, and she is unlikely to want an extended foreplay session. Sex for her at that time of the day is often just another hassle to get through.

How early do the children go to bed? Couldn't you turn the television off some nights, relax for a while, then have sex as part of your time together? If there is a good programme on at 9.30 p.m., you can always switch the television back on again!

If the kids stay up late, can't you go to your bedroom anyway? You can tell them you and your partner need time alone, and if it becomes part of the household routine, it will be accepted without question. Even if they suspect what is going on, I would think they are being reared to see sex as healthy and worth spending time on.

What about the mornings, particularly weekends? It is usually a bad time for a woman who has to get breakfast organised, but perhaps you could encourage your children to be more independent and put a lock on your door so they will not interrupt.

Can you arrange for the children to sleep overnight elsewhere occasionally?

In the end, you must be realistic. If you rarely spend much time relaxing together, you should not expect to have sex very often. Sex should not be a matter of fitting it in whenever you happen to have a spare moment. Generations ago, before electricity, I would think that there was much more time spent on sex because it was an enjoyable pastime and there was not much else to do. Once it got dark and cold, snuggling together was a good way to pass the time, as well as keep warm.

Now we expect it to be wonderful without devoting time to it. And I do not just mean time on foreplay. I mean time together as a couple, doing things together and enjoying each other's company. Then sex would tend to happen when it was appropriate, rather than as a last chore to be performed for the day.

From the woman's point of view, she is unlikely to feel like sex if she is tired, if she is preoccupied with something else (for example, halfway through the washing), if she thinks someone is going to arrive soon, or if she has just been woken up when her partner finishes afternoon shift. It may sound dull, not like in the movies, but since we live in reality we must become more realistic about when we expect ourselves, male or female, to feel like sex. This is particularly true for a woman with low drive, who would much rather go to sleep anyway.

The "where"

The classic scene in the movies is the couple on the beach, making love as the waves gently wash over their bodies.

Whenever I see a scene like that, all I think of is a) they must be cold; b) the sand must be getting in some strange places; c) they are probably getting eaten alive by sandflies and d) what are they going to dry themselves on afterwards?

While it may be romantic to think about making love in unusual places, do not be surprised if neither the man nor the woman is all that keen, particularly if his or her sex drive is usually low.

I mentioned earlier that for some women, pre-marital sex was better than sex after marriage. For other women, though, this is not true if the only place available to have sex is in the car. With wind whistling through the car, the gear stick pressing in the back, bodies tangled so that intercouse requires gymnastic ability, sex in the car can be disastrous, particularly for the woman.

However, just to emphasise the point that sexuality is expressed differently amongst individuals, I recently met a woman who enjoyed sex more in unusual places away from home because she felt she left the daily hassles behind. And there are others who have fond memories of their sexual experiences in cars.

A more common problem for the woman who has been married a few years, is when her bedroom is next to the children's, or they are living with elderly parents. The proximity of the bedrooms often makes a woman embarrassed to have sex in case someone hears. While the man says, "What does it matter?", it is often a real problem for her. If possible, think about insulating the walls, or moving the bed as far as possible to the other side of the room.

Living in a caravan can also put a dampener on a woman's sexual desire, particularly if children are sleeping nearby.

If the woman typically has a low sex drive, she probably will not be too keen to have sex in the bath, or on the kitchen table. I would suggest you put off these ideas for a while.

For a woman who is not that keen on sex, the "where" of sex has to be somewhere she feels comfortable, warm and sure she is not going to be interrupted.

The "why"

As we saw in Chapter 2, many males seem to be endowed with a stronger physical sex drive than women, for a combination of biological and cultural reasons. And with all the cultural emphasis on the physical, exciting side of sex, it seems to have become assumed that the main reason to have sex is physical release. Therefore, by this definition, sex without arousal and orgasm has failed in some way.

Now this puts women at a serious disadvantage, particularly if she has a low physical desire and difficulty with arousal and orgasm.

It also does the male a disservice because women sometimes wrongly assume that they only want sex for physical satisfaction.

We know, in fact, that both men and women seek sex for many different reasons, and we need to become more open about this. Our belief that sex must necessarily be exciting is far too restricting and is one of the reasons why women with low drive avoid sex.

Let's look at it from the woman's point of view if she has low drive. Foreplay usually involves sexual stimulation which may simply irritate her, she does not get aroused so intercourse is often uncomfortable because her vagina is dry, and she rarely if ever comes to orgasm to reward her for her efforts. Naturally she does not look forward to sex.

For this woman, it is necessary to rethink why the couple are having sex, so that she has some reason to want it.

First of all, she needs to realise that most men who care about their partners do not want sex merely for physical release. Men have feelings, too, but because they have been conditioned by society not to be emotional and affectionate, sex becomes their way of saying, "I love you". He wants sex because he cares about his partner; it is just that he is also lucky enough to be able to arouse and enjoy orgasm at the same time. Many men are genuinely distressed by their partner's lack of interest in sex not only because of sexual frustration, but because they feel emotionally rejected.

This is relevant to why you avoid cuddles — because he always wants to follow on with sex. Sure, when you cuddle him, he gets an erection. This is because he feels good. But it does not mean he needs to have sex. Obviously, if it has been quite a while since you had sex, he is going to take the opportunity to try his luck, while you seem to be happy with him. The solution here is not to avoid cuddles, which just means that any cuddle is significant and raises his hopes that *maybe* you feel interested tonight, but to cuddle him as often as possible. If you give him a hug before you go to work, and cuddle him every night before you both go to sleep, and any other time that seems appropriate, he will soon get over the need to try for sex every time, and appreciate cuddles for their own sake.

Your man does not just want to use you sexually, but he may need some help from you to teach him to put less emphasis on the physical side of sex.

The man needs to realise that for the woman with low drive, having sex is a real effort. He should not expect too much from her. He should not feel obliged to try to arouse her. He has to be gentle with his caresses, avoiding the breasts and the genitals if she finds that annoying, and allow her to be passive. He will get more response from her if he makes love to her because he cares about her, and if he appreciates that lying quietly does not mean that she is not enjoying what is happening.

If the woman knows that she can have sex quietly and passively, and that she is not expected to do anything she cannot handle at that time, she is far more likely to agree to have sex. But if she thinks that by agreeing to have sex she is expected to cope with attempts at arousal and orgasm, and put up with things she finds annoying, of course she is not going to be all that interested.

Types A and B women I described earlier need this passive, non-demand sex in the early months of tackling the problem, because they find anything else downright annoying. Once she trusts her partner to try to do the things that please her, she is more likely to relax and gradually become more responsive.

A Type C woman, who can sometimes become aroused and come to orgasm once foreplay has begun, also needs to know that her partner does not always expect her to turn on. This woman is often restricting the times she agrees to sex to those occasions when she is confident she *can* become aroused. This naturally limits the frequency quite a bit, since she certainly does not feel randy every day. If a Type C woman knows that on some occasions she does not have to try to become aroused, but can be passive and just enjoy the sensual contact, then she is likely to agree to sex more often.

Nevertheless, the problem still remains, even for Type C women, that they still never actually feel like sex.

In my experience the only solution to this problem is to think of a frequency that you think you could cope with. Once a week? Once a fortnight? Fine. Then, somewhere in that time period, try to make a conscious decision that now is a reasonable time to have sex. Maybe it is not going to be that great, but then it is not going to be that bad, either. The point is, you are only going to learn to enjoy sex by practice, so avoiding sex for weeks means that nothing is going to change.

This approach depends on trust and communication. The woman needs to be able to trust her partner to allow her to be and respond as she feels at that time, and must be able to communicate to him what makes her feel good or annoyed.

By starting to increase their sexual frequency in this way, provided both partners do not feel angry or resentful about it, they should begin to feel closer and more supportive. As sex becomes more pleasant and enjoyable, the woman is likely to start to look forward to sex, and this is the beginning of the development of sex drive.

Other points to consider

Other factors which may be important in low drive are whether sex is ever painful, whether sex seems messy, whether the woman is turned off by the penis, and whether the woman is using adequate contraception. There may also be other issues I have not mentioned which are relevant to you; do not think they are not important because I have left them out. Discuss the situation with your partner and see if you can come up with your own solutions.

I am going to deal with painful intercourse in detail in Chapter 6. It is obvious that if intercourse hurts, the woman is going to avoid it. The simplest cause of painful intercourse is lack of vaginal lubrication due to lack of arousal. For a woman who is avoiding sex because it hurts, I suggest you try using an artificial lubricant such as K-Y Jelly or baby oil, and see if this helps. If it does, fine. If not, turn to Chapter 6.

A number of women are turned off by the messiness of sex. Here it is, late at night, she has just had a shower and she is feeling warm and clean and snug, and now he wants sex. Or, they made love in the morning, now she has to get up and cook breakfast, and she is feeling rather uncomfortable down below. This is quite reasonable! She should not be embarrassed about it. A box of tissues and either tampons or panty-pads by the bed are a good solution. When they have finished making love, she can put a wad of tissues between her legs rather than jumping up immediately and rushing to the bathroom. Afterplay, when the couple lies contentedly together, is just as important as foreplay, so sometimes it is a pity to break the mood by leaving the bed. If it is time to settle down for the night, she can drop the tissues in a bag by the bed and use the panty-pad or tampon. Tampons are possibly easier, but then some women are put off by the publicity about toxic shock syndrome, so it is up to her. If it is morning, both can take the time to duck in and have a quick shower. It is silly to let a simple thing like this put someone off wanting sex, when if you think logically about it you can come up with a simple solution.

Another common factor in low sex drive is that many women find the sight or touch of the penis somewhat unappealing. Although sex books and movies seem to assume that women should be turned on by the sight of the penis, this is often far from the case. Most females do not get the opportunity to learn to see the male organ as attractive, since the penis is considered offensive and kept out of view. Naked women, however, are on display all over the place: calendars, centrefolds, movies, cards. In our society, it is easy for men to learn that the female body is attractive. For the woman, often the first she sees of a penis, particularly an erect one, is when she starts petting in her teens, and she may well find it somewhat offputting. Some women have quite strong negative feelings about looking at or touching the penis, and this can make them feel reluctant to participate actively in foreplay. Tension and conflict develop if he asks her to touch his penis and she is reluctant to do so. If this is the case with you, take heart that you are not alone. During foreplay over the next few weeks, only do what you can cope with — this might be at best a fleeting touch to the penis. Try to relax about how you feel, don't tell yourself you *must* have a problem to feel this way. Over several months, gradually try to increase the amount of time you can fondle the penis. Eventually, if you proceed at your own pace, you may find that you feel quite friendly towards the penis. However, you may never actually ever be turned on by the sight or touch of the penis, but I don't see that that should be a major problem.

Finally, are you avoiding sex because you are afraid of becoming pregnant? With the current disillusionment with the contraceptive pill, many women are finding that their fertility is not under their control as they had thought. Even if you are using a diaphragm with spermicidal cream, the risk of pregnancy is still higher than with the pill. I would suggest that you make an appointment at the Family Planning Association, or your family general practitioner, to discuss what options are available.

Also, research has shown that the contraceptive pill can decrease sex drive for some women. This is more likely to occur if the woman is taking a pill balanced towards the synthetic hormone progestogen, rather than oestrogen, even if the pill is a low dosage one. Even if the contraceptive pill is not the initial cause of your low drive, it may hinder your progress. It would be worthwhile talking to your doctor about some of the newer sequential-type pills that are available. However, some women don't suit these pills either. And even if a change of pill does help, you will not notice its effects for several months. Nevertheless, the pill does remain the contraceptive of choice for many women, so if it does affect your sex drive but you still want to use it, you may have to be realistic about what you can expect from yourself with regard to your sex drive.

MALE LACK OF DRIVE

It is not nearly as common for a male to experience persistent low sex drive since adolescence, although it can happen. Before I spend any time trying to counsel him, I would ensure that he was thoroughly checked out by a medical practitioner as there may well be a physical cause to his problem.

However, I have seen men whose persistent low sex drive has developed for similar reasons as with a female. He may come from an inhibited sexual background, and never have felt comfortable with sexual issues. It is likely that he did not masturbate, or only rarely, through adolescence. Therefore, like the female, he has not developed his physical sex drive, and has not learnt to use his mind to think erotically to help him look forward to sex. His predicament is often worse than for his female counterpart, because it is so contrary to the common male sexual stereotype. This can cause him considerable distress, depressing any sex drive even further.

If his partner's sexual needs are also low, there may be no major problem in the relationship. But if his partner desires intercourse with any regularity, both can feel extremely depressed and embarrassed by the situation.

It is also more difficult for the male because, whereas a woman can lie back and allow intercourse to happen even if she is not that interested, a man cannot.

Like the woman with low drive, this man has to appreciate that if he wants his sex drive to improve he will only do it gradually and not by pressuring himself. Re-read the previous section for the female with low drive, and try a similar programme yourself. Also, later on in this chapter I will be discussing alternatives to intercourse, which may take some of the pressure off you.

A more common male problem with sex drive is the man who used to have a reasonable sex drive, but in recent months or years finds he is not nearly as keen.

For men with this problem, it is often the case that they are going through a stressful period in their lives, or they have a physical illness. It could also be the result of medication or other drugs (including alcohol) that they are consuming. Although the male sex drive does seem more robust than the female's, nevertheless, if a male feels pressured, ill, depressed or anxious over a period of time, this lack of well-being can certainly decrease his desire for sex. If the stress is going to end at some time in the near future, it is often a case of merely waiting it out. If the stress is likely to continue for some considerable time, the man would be better advised to use his energy to deal with the ongoing problem than to worry about his sex drive. His drive will not pick up while he feels so bad. However, he might find that occasionally he feels a bit more like his old self. Enjoy these episodes, but do not be surprised if next week you return to feeling uninterested as your problems get on top of you again. What you need now is someone who cares about you, and can replace sexual needs with affection and support. Do not avoid physical contact such as cuddles and massage, and sometimes these sessions will develop into sex. However, you will find that you are often quite content to drift into sleep instead.

Another common cause of low desire in the male is when the man has previously had a good sexual relationship that ended some considerable time ago, and he has had no sexual activity, including masturbation, since. Over the last few years his sex drive has gradually decreased, almost, you might say, through lack of practice. Researchers have found that there is a reciprocal relationship between testosterone (the male sex hormone) and sexual activity. Normal levels of testosterone are partly responsible for the man seeking sex regularly. But it seems that regular sexual activity also keeps the testosterone production up in some way. If the man's sexual activity decreases or ceases altogether then testosterone production also decreases, although it may still be within the normal range. This is turn means that the man feels less interested sexually. This slowdown in production of testosterone occurs gradually, so that if the man's sexual activity ceases abruptly, for example if his partner becomes ill, then he will continue to feel sexually frustrated for some time. If sexual outlets continue to be unavailable for several months, however, his sex drive will begin to match his sexual activity.

To develop your sex drive again, you have to get into training! Begin to masturbate once in a while (even though you may feel uncomfortable about this) and, when you develop a new relationship, start at a slow walk rather than trying to launch into a full gallop. I have seen a number of men who have begun a new relationship, trying to have sex once or twice a week and then getting upset with themselves because they are having trouble with arousal. If you have not had regular sexual activity over the last few months or more, you cannot expect yourself to suddenly start functioning at such a level. Have sex only every couple of weeks initially. The woman will usually understand if you talk to her about it. Over a couple of months your sex drive will gradually return to normal.

EXCESSIVE SEX DRIVE

My dictionary defines "excess" as: "that which goes beyond what is usual or necessary; lack of moderation, overindulgence". It is in this sense that I am using the word "excessive".

Although problems with excessive drive do not seem to be as common as complaints of lack of drive, when they do occur they are just as destructive.

Because we live in a society that is hooked on super-sexuality, the person with excessive drive is usually admired, particularly if that person is a male.

Females in the same situation are often considered "slack" or "tramps".

In the cases that I have seen of excessive sex drive, the person, usually male, is unable to be reasonable about his sexual demands. It is irrelevant to him that his partner is tired, or simply does not feel like sex. He considers himself badly done by if he does not have sex at least once a day, sometimes expecting it more often.

I must confess my bias and admit that of all the many and varied sexual problems I have encountered in over a decade of clinical practice, this problem is the *only one* that actually at times makes me feel anger rather than sympathy. This is because, perhaps due to the fact that I am a female, I find it extremely difficult to get through to these men that they *are* being unreasonable, and that *they* have the problem, not their partners. No matter how I approach the problem in the office, when he is at home he continues to pressure his partner to have sex. He refuses to see that his actions are a major cause of the general conflict in the relationship. He usually says that there would not be any problem if his partner would just give him sex, so it is all her fault.

To a lesser degree, the same problem arises when the woman has low sex drive and the man will not moderate his demands to give her some breathing space. As we saw earlier in the chapter, in the initial stages of progress the woman might only want to have intercourse once a fortnight, and any reasonable man (as most are, in my experience) can support his partner in this. Granted, it may not be ideal and he may feel sexually frustrated (see alternatives to intercourse later in the chapter), but I have never known sexual frustration to be fatal.

My own feeling is that excessive sex drive in males is likely to be a symptom of sexual inadequacy, despite what men's magazines would have us believe. A confident, mature male, while he may desire sex every day as an ideal, does not let that override every other consideration in a relationship. If it happens that both partners are happy with sex twice daily or whatever, obviously there is no problem.

Unfortunately, the male with excessive sex drive has to admit to himself that he has a problem before he is prepared to do anything about it. Since I have found this difficult to achieve, I would suggest that the couple see a male sex therapist, or a co-therapy team of a male and a female. If the man is totally unwilling to seek help, then I suggest the woman seek counselling to improve her self-confidence and her assertiveness. Maybe this will give her the encouragement, strength and skills to enable her to express her love to her partner but at the same time stand up to his unreasonable demands.

Where it is the woman that has an excessive sex drive, there seem to be two major possible causes. The first is that demonstrated by researchers such as Marc Hollender, who found that women often initiate sex out of a need to be held and cuddled rather than for sex *per se*. The other common cause is when the woman is desperately trying to learn to orgasm, and is badgering her partner to practise at every opportunity. Unfortunately, the harder she tries the less likely she is to orgasm, and the more frustrated she becomes.

In the case of the first woman, she needs to come to understand why she so desperately seeks affection, and to learn more appropriate ways of developing relationships. Again, counselling aimed at improving self-esteem and assertive behaviour should be helpful. You could ask your family doctor to suggest a qualified therapist for you to consult.

The woman who is desperately trying to learn to orgasm might find Chapter 7 helpful.

INCOMPATIBLE SEX DRIVES

This section will deal with the situation where neither partner could be considered to have a problem with drive, but their sex drives simply do not match up very well. Some of the suggestions will also be useful for people who are experiencing specific problems with drive.

With some couples, the normal fluctuation in desire over the years which encompasses the various life events such as child-raising, financial difficulties and so on, means that sometimes their sex drives match, while at other times one or the other has the greater interest. This is all quite normal and should not cause undue worry about the rest of their relationship.

What we are looking for in the situation of mismatched sex drives, is compromise. This also applies to well-matched couples if on any particular occasion one is boiling with frustration and the other is totally disinterested.

Step number one involves recognising:
a) that it is reasonable that you feel the way *you* do; and

b) it is reasonable that your partner feels the way she or he does.

It should not be a cause of conflict, merely a minor clash of interests to be sorted out.

Then it is a matter of looking for alternatives to compromise, and it is here that some of you may not approve. If you do not feel any of the suggestions are appropriate for you, leave them and if possible work out other suitable compromises with your partner.

Think about how you feel about masturbation, whether it is yourself or your partner, because the most obvious alternative to intercourse is self-stimulation. I see this as quite reasonable, but I realise that many people still do not feel comfortable with it.

However, when a person with a normal sex drive does not have the opportunity for intercourse, masturbation is a convenient solution. I know that in some relationships this is done with a lot of secrecy, but I feel it is better if possible to be able to discuss it with your partner.

So, if your partner feels sexy and you don't, it seems reasonable that she or he masturbate to relieve sexual frustration. However, it is infinitely more satisfying if you can support what your partner is doing by putting your head on his or her shoulder, or caressing the chest, tickling the thighs, or whatever feels nice. In this way you are acknowledging that you are with your partner in spirit, if not in body.

The other alternative is for you to arouse and bring your partner to orgasm manually. This is fine if you are not feeling too tired, otherwise, not only can it be a pain in the neck so to speak, but a pain in the hand, arm, shoulder and back as well. Bringing someone to orgasm by hand, while pleasurable to the receiver, is often hard work for the doer. But if you are not too tired and you have your sense of humour intact, it can be a lot of fun. Just make sure you are in a comfortable position before you begin.

Another alternative is mutual manual stimulation which is nice for those lazy occasions when you both feel that an orgasm would be nice but one or both of you cannot be bothered doing too much work. The position I suggest is that you both lie on your backs, side by side, your feet next to your partner's head. Both put your nearest arm underneath your partner's nearest leg, which is raised slightly. This then gives you comfortable, easy access to your partner's nether regions. This position is also convenient when only one partner feels the need for orgasm; the other can lie there thinking about all sorts of irrelevant things, quite comfortable while the other partner enjoys the stimulation.

It is also worthwhile considering acquiring a vibrator. The best ones are not the penis-shaped type, but body massagers which have a flat rubber pad for massage of the face. The vibrator can be used by either male or female, and provided the person feels comfortable using it, it can produce an orgasm without too much effort. For this reason it is a handy alternative when one partner feels sexy and the other doesn't. The vibrator can be used by the partner or by the person himself (or herself), and it is worthwhile experimenting with it to see what feels good.

There are obviously also going to be occasions

when the compromise needs to be in the interests of the partner who is simply too tired, tense or whatever to even consider sexual interaction. Then the sexy partner may simply have to be satisfied with a cuddle.

In the end, the ability to compromise through caring and consideration will determine the outcome of any situation in which the individual needs of the couple differ.

5 PROBLEMS WITH PERFORMANCE
Part I: The Male

While problems with drive are more common amongst females, most male problems fall into the performance category.

PREMATURE EJACULATION

In my opinion this particular problem is given far too much attention. It is emphasised out of all proportion to its importance.

First of all, let us consider what premature ejaculation is. It has been variously defined as the inability of the male to withhold ejaculation to enable the woman to orgasm at least 50 per cent of the time (provided she is able to orgasm with intercourse); or to withhold ejaculation for longer than 60 seconds after penetration.

The initial cause of premature ejaculation may be due to the fact that as an adolescent, the male would try to orgasm as quickly as possible during masturbation because of guilt or fear of being caught; or to anxiety during initial attempts at intercourse which set the pattern for rapid ejaculation; or a period of stress which triggered premature ejaculation initially but then continues after the stress has ended; and so on.

Whatever the initial cause of the problem, it is being maintained by anxiety. For the male, negative feelings, such as tiredness and worry, typically cause ejaculation to occur more rapidly. By always being anxious whenever he has sex (will it happen again?) the male automatically ensures that premature ejaculation will continue to happen. Over a period of time, premature ejaculation becomes an established habit.

Before we discuss suggestions for dealing with premature ejaculation, however, we need to put rapid ejaculation into perspective.

Firstly, the male needs to be reassured that rapid ejaculation (I prefer that term) under stress makes sense when we consider the biological purpose of intercourse. Going back to the dim dark days of our cavemen ancestors, it was essential that the male be able to finish intercourse by rapid ejaculation if a huge mammoth or whatever suddenly came charging towards the entwined couple. Obviously males who could not ejaculate under the many and varied stresses to which primitive man was subjected would be less likely to impregnate females. Therefore males who could ejaculate rapidly under stress would tend to predominate in terms of genetic inheritance. So rapid ejaculation has a natural basis.

Secondly, many men who are convinced they are premature ejaculators are often functioning quite normally — ejaculating one to six minutes after penetration. Occasional success at delaying intercourse for 10 minutes or more does not mean that you should always be able to do this. If you want to practise delaying ejaculation for hours, as some sexual philosophies suggest, fine, but I do not see that as being a prerequisite to being a good lover. You are doing fine if you ejaculate only a couple of minutes after entry, disappointing though that may sound compared to the super-feats of the heroes of fiction.

Thirdly, sometimes premature ejaculation is due to his anxiety that if only he could last longer, she would orgasm with penile thrusting. Many women require 10 minutes or more of penile thrusting to achieve orgasm. This sounds like a lot of hard work to me if it is a regular demand or expectation. Rather than treating the rapid ejaculation brought about by the male's anxiety at having to perform so well all the time, I feel it is more reasonable to encourage the couple to be more flexible in their sexual expectations. The ideal of prolonged penile thrusting resulting in orgasm is unlikely to occur unless both partners are relaxed and feeling good. So reserve it for those occasions, and take the pressure off both of you. Try other alternatives such as mutual masturbation, self-stimulation by the female during intercourse, orgasm during foreplay, vibrators, and so on, to reduce the need for the male to delay ejaculation on most occasions. Sex that has become hard work is no fun at all, and will only mean that the male's "premature" ejaculation is likely to continue indefinitely.

Fourthly, if you and your partner enjoy extended foreplay, then you are obviously going to be highly aroused and ready to ejaculate when intercourse occurs. Therefore, you should not be surprised when ejaculation happens quickly. Also if you and your partner have infrequent sex, you are going to be very sensitive to any sexual stimulation when it does occur, so again rapid ejaculation under those circumstances would be quite normal. Similarly, if you are going through a stressful period of your life you must realistically expect to have less control over ejaculation.

Lastly, the value of rapid ejaculation seems to be overlooked. Given, as I have said earlier, that the male sex drive is often higher than the female, and given that she does not always want to arouse and come to orgasm, many women enjoy the fact that at least on some occasions their partners ejaculate rapidly. He often believes that his partner is disappointed, and she is often reluctant to tell him that actually his rapid ejaculation sometimes suits her. When he stops worrying about what his partner thinks, he is likely to be able to delay ejaculation a little longer anyway, and she often is not that fussed to have him delay it for 10 minutes or so. You and your partner should discuss what suits both of you, rather than trying to live up to some arbitrary standard of success which might suit neither of you. For many couples, foreplay is more important than intercourse itself, so it makes more sense to spend your energy there rather than wearing yourself out in intercourse.

The treatment

If you are ejaculating very rapidly and would still like to do something about it, you might try the following suggestions.

Before you begin, talk to your partner about how you feel about your ejaculatory pattern. Sometimes the woman is making the problem worse by being scornful or angry, or even by being too sympathetic. She needs to understand her role in your progress. If she is antagonistic or patronising, you are going to continue to feel tense during foreplay so that rapid ejaculation will almost certainly continue to occur. If she is too sympathetic, this is going to over-emphasise the rapid ejaculation at the expense of relaxing and enjoying foreplay. She needs to be supportive and caring, and be prepared for gradual rather than immediate improvement.

Then, you must accept that, at least for the next several weeks, you are going to continue to ejaculate rapidly. Stop pressuring yourself to solve your problem immediately, and start to relax. There is no point in being angry with yourself whenever you do not delay ejaculation. This will only make you more tense and more likely to maintain the problem. Also, do not avoid sexual contact because of fear or embarrassment that you might "fail". Infrequent ejaculation will make you more sensitive when sexual stimulation does occur, again making it likely that you will ejaculate quickly.

For the first couple of weeks you might like to substitute masturbation for intercourse. If you masturbate on your own, you can use these sessions as practice in relaxing and enjoying the stimulation prior to orgasm. This is the reverse of what you probably did as a teenager, when you tried to come as quickly as possible.

The problem for many men actually begins during foreplay, when they begin to anticipate "failure". Initially you need to forget about intercourse and learn to enjoy foreplay. Practise your fantasising, enjoy thinking sexy thoughts instead of worrying about your performance. If you find it hard to think up a nice, sexy fantasy, begin by focusing on your partner's hands as she caresses your body, and mentally say to yourself: "That feels nice, that feels really good." This helps you to appreciate the present rather than worry about the future. If it suits you both, bring your partner to orgasm during foreplay so that there is no pressure to delay ejaculation if you do decide to have intercourse. However, it would probably be less stressful if you both came to orgasm with mutual masturbation, vibrator, or whatever, in the initial stages of treatment.

If you do decide to have intercourse, relax and enjoy your orgasm no matter how rapidly ejaculation occurs. As you relax in anticipation of orgasm, you are much more likely to delay ejaculation. But it may take several weeks to change your habitual ejaculatory pattern, so do not expect too much too soon.

Some men like to use a condom during intercourse to decrease sensitivity. If this is acceptable to both partners it is worth a try. Similarly, some men use a mild anaesthetic cream that is available from most pharmacies. If these methods are used it should only be for a short time until the man feels more relaxed and confident. After a while he should try intercourse again without these aids.

Some men try during intercourse to think about non-sexual things such as counting backwards from 100 in order to feel less aroused. Some even bite their cheeks or do other painful and distracting things to decrease arousal and delay orgasm. In my opinion these methods are a waste of time, since they make sex hard work and less enjoyable.

Sometimes tensing the muscles of the bottom during intercourse is a simple and unobtrusive method of delaying orgasm. Though it is not completely clear why this works it appears that this action interferes with the normal physiological changes in the genital area that precede orgasm.

In a similar vein, a method known as the Beautrais manoeuvre can also be useful. This technique makes use of the fact that, prior to ejaculation, the man's testicles ascend to cling to the base of the penis. For a man who is ready to ejaculate on penetration, his testicles will already have ascended. So, before penetration, he should reach behind and gently pull his testicles down away from the base of the penis. With practice, he can also perform this manoeuvre during intercourse whenever he would like to delay ejaculation. It is worth experimenting to find the most comfortable way of performing the Beautrais manoeuvre.

Recently there has also been some suggestion that ejaculatory control can be improved if the man exercises the muscles of the pelvic floor. Although these exercises were originally designed for women, it now seems that if a man practises the first two exercises given on page 195 on a daily basis, he will also notice some benefits resulting from improved muscle tone. During intercourse, he may then be able to delay ejaculation simply by tensing the pelvic floor.

If these simple suggestions do not help, then you can consider using the squeeze technique. This requires the help of a sympathetic partner, and regular practice.

The first stage involves the woman sitting on the bed, resting comfortably against the bedhead, while the man lies on his back facing her with his buttocks between her spread legs, and his genital area as near to her as possible so that she can comfortably handle his penis.

Using a little oil or hand cream, she stimulates his penis with her hand. When the man feels he is about to ejaculate he indicates this to her, and she quickly but firmly squeezes the penis, using two fingers and a thumb, at the point where the head meets the shaft

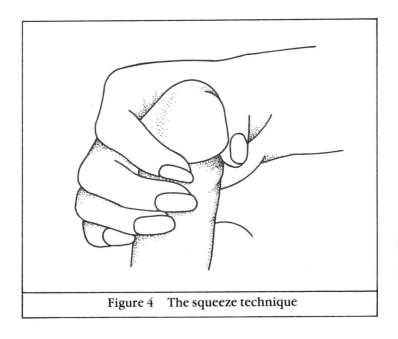

Figure 4   The squeeze technique

(Figure 4). The two fingers are placed on the stomach side of the penis, and the thumb on the other. The squeeze, which will cause the desire to ejaculate to subside, is maintained for about five seconds, then both partners relax for about a minute. Stimulation of the penis is then resumed and, as before, when ejaculation is imminent the squeeze is reapplied. This is repeated seven or eight times, then ejaculation is allowed to take place.

By repeating these sessions on a daily basis, if possible, in a short time a pattern of sexual response can be established in which the man is able to tolerate intense stimulation yet delay ejaculation. He is then ready to try intercourse.

After relaxing foreplay, with cuddles and massage, he enters her, but instead of thrusting, stays still and quiet within her. Initially, the woman-on-top position may be a good idea. She may need to use lubrication around the vagina, and then insert the penis as she straddles her partner. After a short time, if he feels in control, the woman can slowly begin to move, while he enjoys every sensation of pleasure, not worrying when he might ejaculate. If he feels that ejaculation is going to occur before he wants it to, he indicates to his partner to stop moving and remain still till the feeling subsides. The control gained by the squeeze technique should mean that the man takes longer to ejaculate than previously.

After a few sessions with the woman on top, the couple can then try the man-on-top position. Again, the same principles of stop-start are applied. With repeated practice he can gradually extend his time to ejaculation. However, during this programme he will at times ejaculate rapidly as before. This is quite normal so do not give up. Continue to practise with the squeeze technique until you are confident once more of greater control. Ultimately you should be able to have intercourse spontaneously and ejaculate normally without any special effort.

IMPOTENCE

While I believe premature ejaculation to be a somewhat overrated sexual problem, impotence, that is, difficulties in obtaining and maintaining an erection, can be quite devastating.

For centuries, the erect penis has been a symbol of masculinity, and the male who finds himself unable to have an erection can suffer feelings of embarrassment, shame, anxiety and a sense of loss of masculinity.

It is this emotional reaction to erectile dysfunction that is, in fact, the main stumbling block in the treatment of impotence.

The initial causes of impotence are many and varied. Most men experience occasional problems which are of no significance. Too much alcohol, fatigue, or worry, can all mean that on a particular occasion a man will be unable to achieve an erection.

For some men, the difficulty can last for several weeks, months or even years.

We need to distinguish between two major categories of impotence. The first category, *primary impotence*, refers to those men who have *never* been able to achieve an erection sufficient to perform intercourse. The second category, *secondary impotence*, refers to those men who at some stage previously could successfully have intercourse, but are having difficulty now.

For men with primary impotence, the initial cause is likely to be either that they had a disastrous first attempt at intercourse, or they felt uncomfortable and embarrassed by sexual matters. I recall one young man, for example, who was interrupted by his father during his first attempt at intercourse, and his embarrassment related to that incident precipitated several years of unsuccessful attempts. Another young man came from a sexually inhibited family. He had avoided masturbation as much as possible and was generally uncomfortable making sexual overtures to a woman, and, consequently, had never been able to become aroused with one.

For men with secondary impotence, the initial episode is usually caused by a situational problem such as financial worry, marital conflict, illness, abuse of alcohol, and so on. Often these men fail to connect their erectile problem with its cause, so they begin to worry about their sexuality as well as the other problem.

It is important to note that there are also possible physical causes of impotence, including injury, illness, medication, disease, drug abuse and abnormal hormone production. Our understanding of the physiology of erection is still incomplete, and it can sometimes be very difficult for the cause of an individual's impotence to be clearly defined. For example, some men can ejaculate and experience orgasm although they only have a partial erection. Others might awaken with an erection but not be able to obtain an erection under any other circumstances. The cause in these cases may be either physical or psychological or a combination of both. Therefore it is advisable that any man who experiences difficulties with erection be thoroughly checked out by a medical specialist who is specifically interested in problems relating to erectile dysfunction. However, if a man can successfully achieve an erection during masturbation, or with one partner but not another, it is highly unlikely that there is a physical cause of the problem.

If there is a physical problem, then you must rely on your doctor's advice for treatment. Sometimes the physical problem is such that the man is unlikely to be able to have erections again. If this turns out to be the case with you, try not to throw up your hands in despair. It may be possible for you to have implanted into your penis a device that allows you to artificially erect the penis. However, not all cases are suitable for this procedure, so it may be that you and your partner have to build your sex lives around the fact that you cannot achieve a good erection. It will take a special relationship with your partner to deal with this, but it can be done. Lack of erection does not have to mean the end of physical intimacy. Some men can still ejaculate despite no erection. Experiment with what you can do. Do not avoid cuddles, massage, and other alternatives such as masturbation and oral sex. It is fair enough to be upset that your sex life has been permanently changed, but it is not reasonable to allow this to destroy your relationship with your partner.

I would like to mention at this stage that over the years there has been a number of research studies which link smoking to impotence in some cases. Smoking is known to affect the vascular (blood vessels) system in some cases, by clogging it in different places. Some researchers claim that the blood vessels which supply the penis can be affected in this way, making it difficult for the penis to engorge with blood during arousal. The good news is that giving up smoking may well improve the situation. This must be the ultimate incentive to give up smoking!

Another factor, which is often overlooked in the case of the man who has difficulty maintaining an erection during intercourse, is whether the woman's vagina is providing enough stimulation to keep the man aroused. Often, if the woman has had children, her vaginal muscles may have lost some of their tone. If this is the case, it would help if the woman started practising the vaginal exercises found on page 195. This should also help her receive more enjoyment from intercourse. In other instances, the man feels that the woman becomes too wet, making the vagina extremely slippery and therefore reducing grip. Unfortunately, however, I haven't come across any good solution to this problem, except to suggest that they use a tissue to wipe the excess lubrication from her vagina just prior to entry.

If physical causes seem unlikely, then irrespective of whether the man has primary or secondary impotence, a major factor in the ongoing difficulty with erection is the man's anxiety over his sexual performance and his fear of failure.

Continuing strife in the relationship, financial difficulties or emotional problems, such as depression, can maintain impotence for weeks or months. If and when these causes are removed, the man's ability to achieve an erection should return. Unfortunately, many men often do not realise that their problems have realistic causes. Therefore, instead of accepting the situation with frustrated resignation, they begin to worry. In our society we place so much emphasis on sexual success that it is very difficult for a man to remain calm in the face of what is thought of as a failure.

It is this worry about failure that maintains the man's problems for long after the end of the original stress. Whenever the man considers having sex he is almost immediately beset by the thought: "What if it happens again?" This thought stays with him during foreplay, when he needs to feel confident and relaxed in order to become aroused. Some men can maintain a good erection during foreplay, but it quickly diminishes at the thought of initiating intercourse. Others get, at best, a partial erection.

Each "failure" reinforces his anxiety about his performance and ultimately some men avoid sex altogether. But this is not the way to overcome the problem. Impotence can be treated; it just takes patience and understanding.

In order to decide what is the best way to treat your particular problem, we need to know the answers to a few questions.

Do you have a regular partner? If you do not have a steady partner it is obviously much more difficult for you to try to overcome your impotence, because you are naturally going to feel embarrassed with each woman with whom you attempt intercourse. You have a couple of options. One is to be honest with your next female friend and sound her out as to how she would feel cooperating with you over the next few weeks to solve your problem. You could also try to find a professional sex surrogate, a woman who is prepared to practise sex with you for a fee. Unfortunately, such professionals are few and far between. A third option is for you to learn to spend time on foreplay, developing your techniques of arousing and satisfying a woman, so that when you are next with a woman who wants to have sex with you, you are confident that you can satisfy her whether or not you get an erection. If you do not get an erection, try to pass it off lightly ("too much booze") and continue to cuddle and/or arouse her until she is satisfied. She may be content not to be aroused, or she may be happy to come to orgasm with manual or oral stimulation. When you feel confident about your ability to please a woman, you should start to relax with women and ultimately become aroused yourself.

If you have a regular partner, is she interested in helping you overcome your impotence? If you have a partner but she is uninterested in your problem (sometimes the woman may even be relieved by it), your situation is also difficult. Indeed, the actual cause of your impotence may well be related to your

wider sexual and/or marital relationship, and you
need to talk to her about this. You may even consider counselling to help you resolve these difficulties. But if your partner is totally uninterested in
improving your sexual relationship, realistically it
seems that you are not in a good position to overcome your impotence. You will not be able to relax
and arouse if you and your partner are tense and
hostile with one another.

If your partner does care about you and wants to
help, do you worry that you are letting her down
when you do not get an erection? Many men do,
usually quite unnecessarily. Since women are quite
capable of being orgasmic during foreplay, they are
not as worried about intercourse as you might think.
Also, many women enjoy the affection and
emotional intimacy rather than the arousal and
orgasm, so again she is more likely to be worried for
your sake than her own. If your partner does need
intercourse to become aroused, you need to discuss
this. If you are both prepared to be patient and
follow the suggested programme, there is a good
chance that over the next few months you will both
be able to be satisfied. In any event, talk to your
partner; do not make yourself miserable imagining
what she may or may not be thinking.

When you do not get an erection, do you get
yourself upset, and either roll over in despair or get
angry and leave the room? If so, this is merely pro-
longing your problem by making each sexual session
more and more tense.

Step number one in the treatment programme is
that, at least for the time being, you must accept as

calmly as possible that you are likely to have trouble having an erection, and try to relax and enjoy foreplay despite this. If you cannot have intercourse, then relax and enjoy the cuddles instead. I realise this is very hard for you to do, but the more complacent you become, the greater your chance of progress. Also, if you have been avoiding any sexual or physical contact with your partner, this is merely adding to the tension.

The second step in the treatment programme is for you and your partner to cuddle and touch often, so that you learn to relax 'with each other. By avoiding contact, there is going to be more tension and strain when you finally do get together.

Now we need to know what you do, think and feel during foreplay. Some men are able to participate in and enjoy foreplay, becoming erect quite easily, and their problem begins only when they think about initiating intercourse. If this is your problem, it is quite easy to treat. All you need to realise is that you have a problem for only the minute or so before and during attempted penetration, when you switch your mind from sexy thoughts to worry: "Will it happen again?" Practise focusing your mind on sexual thoughts, or on your partner's breasts, or on how nice your penis feels against your partner's vagina, and you will find that this will easily enable you to maintain your erection sufficiently to penetrate your partner's vagina.

For the man who is unable to arouse at all, or only slightly during foreplay, you and your partner need to agree not to attempt intercourse at all for the next six weeks. You need to use that time to get together a couple of times a week, cuddling, touching, talking, bringing her to orgasm if she desires. She can touch your penis, but only for your enjoyment, not to see whether you can have an erection or not. If you do happen to get an erection, you *must not* attempt intercourse during the agreed period. In this first stage we are not concerned about whether or not you get an erection since we already know that you have some problem. We are concerned about you learning to relax and to be able to think sexually again. Conjure up all those images that you used to be able to do so easily years ago. Lie back and appreciate the feel of your partner's fingers on your body, your penis. *This* is what you are missing out on in your obsession to have a good erection!

During this stage, it is most helpful if the woman feels comfortable being active with caresses, cuddles and touching. Some women are embarrassed to touch the penis, so talk to her about how she feels. It can be difficult for you to become aroused without such stimulation. Show her or tell her how you like to be touched and ask her about her preferences. Learning to communicate without embarrassment will help you both to have a more enjoyable sexual relationship.

The whole point of this stage is for you to learn not to start on that very destructive train of thought: "Will I fail again?" This is the key to your whole problem. You simply have to replace that unpleasant thought with enjoyable thoughts such as erotic images, or appreciation of what is happening to your body.

I say "simply". It is a simple process, but it is a gradual one. You and your partner must be prepared to proceed slowly. It takes time to break your old habitual way of thinking with a new, more enjoyable pattern. This is why you should not attempt intercourse for at least six weeks. During that time you may well notice that you are starting to get erections, but again it will take time for you to develop the habit of easily developing good erections. So, do not pressure yourself — you have been doing that for quite long enough already! Relax, take it easy, enjoy yourself — time enough to proceed to intercourse later.

If, at the end of six weeks, you have experienced good erections on several occasions, you may decide to try intercourse. But if you have not had an erection, you need to extend stage one for another three weeks. You might also like to consider practising with masturbation. Sometimes the presence of a partner adds to the man's tension and makes relaxation and arousal less likely. So, by practising on your own, you can often learn to relax more easily. Then, by focusing on erotic thoughts, erections occur more spontaneously. When you are more confident about your ability to have an erection, then go back to practising with relaxation and arousal with your partner.

When you are ready to try intercourse, remember that you are likely to lose some arousal. This is quite reasonable. Do not shorten foreplay merely to rush to use your erection. Take it slowly, relax during foreplay. If you get a good erection, fine. If it subsides somewhat, it will come back. Every male notices that his erection develops and subsides during foreplay, so it is a normal process. If your erection disappears, and you cannot relax and allow it to come back, put aside any thought of intercourse for that session and continue with cuddles, talking and so on. This is likely to happen on several occasions over the next few weeks, so do not panic, and keep trying when you feel ready.

You might find it easier in your initial attempts at intercourse if you use the woman-on-top position. You lie back, doing nothing but enjoying those wonderful fantasies in your head, while your partner guides your penis into her vagina with her hands. It might help if she moistens her vagina with some lubrication if she is not aroused. Again, if you lose your erection before entry is achieved, don't keep trying for too long. Your partner can come and lie beside you again, and try again another time.

Another comfortable position to try is the pregnancy, or non-demand, position. After foreplay, both lie on your sides, you facing your partner's back almost at right angles, or whatever is comfortable. Your partner can help guide your penis into her vagina for a leisurely session.

There is no reason why you cannot overcome your impotence over the next few months if you follow this programme, and are content to take things slowly. Just remember, you have to learn how to *allow* your penis to become erect, you cannot *make* it do so. The whole point of the programme is relaxation and enjoyment of all aspects of love-making, not just erection and intercourse.

I want to give special mention again to the man

who is resuming sexual activity after several months or years of abstinence. I discussed this particular case in the section on low drive, but it is worth repeating that if a man has had little or no sexual activity for an extended period of time, he is quite naturally likely to experience some difficulty with arousal when he initiates a new sexual relationship. He must be realistic. He cannot suddenly expect his body to be able to perform two or three times a week. Take it slowly, and do not try to have sex every time you are with your new friend. Begin to practise mastur-bation. This will help to develop your sex drive again, as well as give you confidence that you are quite capable of erection.

Finally, if you are trying to overcome impotence, you must look at what else is happening in your life at the same time. If you have just lost your job, or you and your partner are hassling over some problems, or one of your children is quite ill, stay in stage one of the programme until the pressures ease up. If you have progressed to the intercourse stage and stresses develop in your life, do not be surprised if you are not as successful as you were a week or so ago. Go back to stage one of the programme, enjoying foreplay-type stimulation, and let your penis take care of itself.

RETARDED EJACULATION

This is a less common problem than either premature ejaculation or impotence, but to those men who experience it, it is just as important.

Retarded ejaculation, or ejaculatory incompetence, refers to the difficulty, or inability, of the male to ejaculate during intercourse despite prolonged thrusting. Some men experience this problem on the odd occasion when they have achieved an erection even though they have had far too much to drink; despite their erection, they simply cannot ejaculate due to the depressing effects of the alcohol.

When retarded ejaculation occurs with most or all sexual encounters, it is usually caused by inhibition or embarrassment about sexual matters, by relationship problems, or even by prolonged use of the withdrawal method of contraception which has trained the man to overcontrol his ejaculatory reflex. In some instances, as an adolescent the man might have been embarrassed by or ashamed of his sexual development, and tried to avoid masturbation as an immoral or abnormal thing to do. During masturbation he may well have tried not to dwell on erotic images, almost tried to pretend he was not aroused. This pattern of masturbation would have taught him not to enjoy arousal, even to deny it, and this has established the problem in adulthood. He is unable to relax and enjoy his sexuality, and cannot conjure up sexual images in his mind to enable ejaculation to occur.

In some instances there is the possibility that this problem may have a physical cause, so it is worthwhile having a check-up with a medical practitioner. However, retarded ejaculation is probably more likely to be due to the sort of causes already mentioned.

Usually, the first place to start in the treatment of

this problem, as with so many sexual problems, is with masturbation. It is easier to learn to relax and let go on your own, without the added pressure of your partner being present. It may be difficult for you to give yourself permission to masturbate, and you are very likely going to feel embarrassed, but keep in mind that you do want to be able to enjoy your sex life. Buy yourself some sexy magazines, go and see some R-rated movies. Appreciating these things does not mean you are some sort of pervert; it is quite healthy to enjoy this type of sexual fantasy. You need to develop the ability to enjoy sex with your mind, so that your control of your physical sexuality will lessen.

When you can successfully masturbate to ejaculation on your own, if your partner is agreeable, use self-stimulation during foreplay with her. She can also stimulate you if you find that arousing. When you feel you are close to orgasm, your partner can straddle you for the woman-on-top position, and while you continue self-stimulation, she helps you insert the penis. You can continue to add hand stimulation to the base of the penis as intercourse proceeds, and at the same time continue thinking those sexy thoughts. Sometimes your partner can try to bring you to orgasm manually while you relax and enjoy your fantasies, or play with her body. If you find it difficult to make the step from hand stimulation to intercourse, allow yourself to ejaculate first, then enter the vagina immediately, again preferably using the woman-on-top position. When you can do that easily, have your partner guide the penis into her vagina as you ejaculate with self-stimulation.

Obviously the next step then is that you signal to your partner when ejaculation is imminent, and she inserts the penis just before ejaculation. As you become more confident that you can let go and ejaculate within the vagina, you can spend less time on self-stimulation during foreplay and more time on other techniques, inserting the penis whenever you want.

As with all other sexual problems, you must take your time, because progress may be gradual. Be prepared to go back a step in the programme if stresses develop in your life. Also, the success of the programme depends on the cooperation of your partner and how well you can communicate, so spend time talking about what is happening and how you both feel. And, solving your ejaculation problem is not the full solution to your sexual problem — learning to enjoy your sexuality, to feel relaxed with physical and emotional intimacy, is also important. So, as with premature ejaculation and impotence, spend time on learning to appreciate foreplay and afterplay rather than concentrating only on intercourse.

PAINFUL INTERCOURSE

Some males experience pain during or after intercourse. This is much more likely to be a medical rather than a psychological problem, so I recommend a visit to your medical practitioner.

6 PROBLEMS WITH PERFORMANCE

Part II: The female

Problems with performance experienced by the female fall into two categories, vaginismus and painful intercourse.

VAGINISMUS

This refers to the inability of the vagina to relax and allow penetration by the penis. Like impotence, it can be divided into two categories, primary and secondary.

With *primary vaginismus*, the woman has never been able to permit intercourse to occur. It is more common than is realised for a woman to be married for several months or even years and not to have properly consummated the marriage.

As with other sexual problems, the woman's problem has to be clarified before a decision can be made about treatment. A medical examination is helpful, although of course many women suffering from vaginismus simply cannot relax to allow this to take place. With primary vaginismus, the cause is more likely to be psychological, but this does not rule out the possibility of some physical difficulty which would require medical intervention.

The initial cause of primary vaginismus varies. It

may be that the woman, as an adolescent, was influenced by our cultural preoccupation with pain on first intercourse. Novels abound with detailed descriptions of the seduction of virgins, always including mention of the "cry of pain" she inevitably emits. As a result, many young women approach their first intercourse with trepidation. This anxiety leads to lack of lubrication, tension of the vaginal muscles and, bingo, pain! Therefore, the young woman approaches the next and subsequent attempts with the same anxiety, and chronic vaginismus takes over.

Perhaps surprisingly, a number of young women whom I have seen with this background to their problem actually functioned quite well in all other aspects of their sexuality. Such a woman is aware of her sex drive, enjoys all manner of foreplay, and often can come to orgasm by one means or another. She is likely to feel comfortable bringing her husband to orgasm manually or orally. But she simply cannot allow the penis to enter her vagina. For this woman, the treatment programme is quite simple, although progress is often slow.

For other cases of vaginismus, however, the cause can be quite complex. As we have seen before, if a woman is revolted or sickened by the thought of sex, she is advised to seek individual counselling if she finds this book unhelpful.

In other cases, the cause may be due to general sexual inhibition, perhaps due to inappropriate sex education. It may be due to the fact that she and her partner do not appreciate the differences between male and female sexuality, and so are trying to arouse her in ways that only annoy her. Therefore, when intercourse is attempted the vagina is dry and tense, and intercourse is impossible. Such a woman (and her partner) would be advised to read Chapter 4 first, before attempting to deal with the vaginismus. It may also be due at least in part to poor communication and lack of intimacy in the relationship, so Chapter 8 may be helpful.

When the problem is *secondary vaginismus*, the causes are likely to be somewhat different. With secondary vaginismus the woman has, at one time, been able to successfully allow penetration by the penis, and now, for some reason, she cannot.

A common cause here, initially, is a physical problem. For example, the woman may have had a chronic vaginal infection, or she may have tender scar tissue following childbirth, or she may be chronically fatigued due to some ongoing stress and so fails to lubricate adequately. Whatever the specific reason, the woman experiences pain during intercourse or attempted intercourse for a significant period of time. This causes her to *anticipate* pain whenever she thinks about intercourse. This anticipation leads to anxiety, which sets off the now familiar lack of lubrication/vaginal muscle tension/pain cycle. Therefore, even when the initial cause has disappeared, the woman continues to experience pain with attempted intercourse.

Sometimes, however, the initial physical problem has not been diagnosed and treated, so that the woman may be experiencing pain even though adequately lubricated. I will be dealing with this more fully in the next section on painful intercourse.

As with primary vaginismus, the woman with secondary vaginismus may enjoy all other aspects of sexuality and merely be unable to permit intercourse, or she may avoid all sexual contact.

This last problem often develops because of her fear of attempted intercourse. She may figure that if she allows her partner to caress and cuddle her, it is going to lead to attempts at intercourse, so she avoids that type of intimacy. Then she feels that if she allows her partner even to put his arm around her, it will lead to cuddles and thence to attempts at intercourse. Some women I have seen with either primary or secondary vaginismus had reached the point where they avoided *any* physical contact at all for fear of what it might lead to. No wonder both partners were miserable by the time they came for help.

What to do

Stage I: First of all you need to decide whether your problem is confined only to being unable to permit penetration but you usually enjoy foreplay. If this is the case, you can go straight to Stage II.

However, if you cannot relax even during foreplay, I want you and your partner to agree to ban all attempts at intercourse for the next four weeks.

Instead, in that time you need to agree to have regular cuddle sessions, times when you talk, caress, touch and generally try to relax with one another. If the male is sexually frustrated, he could consider alternative methods of orgasm such as self-stimulation, or manual stimulation by the woman. However, since some vaginismic women are having trouble coming to terms with female sexuality, let alone male sexuality, you may feel uncomfortable manually arousing your partner.

Sometimes the man feels angry, resentful about his partner's inability to have intercourse. He has reached the end of his ability to cope. Therefore, asking him to give even more now may seem too much to ask. But, if he is committed to the relationship, I can only say that it is worthwhile persevering for a little longer. Insisting on continued attempts at intercourse will only end in disaster. If the relationship breaks down as a result of this problem, the woman can still benefit from the programme outlined below.

In the four weeks for which intercourse is banned, you are aiming only for relaxation. Do not worry about arousal. If you have never come to orgasm, you can worry about that later. Now you caress each other gently, emphasising your feelings, enjoying lying quietly and appreciating the tender touch from your partner. Close your eyes, think about how nice it feels to be close, secure.

Try to get into the habit of holding hands when you are out, and give each other a cuddle and kiss when you leave and come home. There is no reason to avoid this now, as intercourse is banned for the time being.

Stage II: On page 195 you will find a set of vaginal exercises. I want you to start practising these daily. They are easy to do and only take a few minutes. They will teach you control of your vaginal muscles and so are an important part of the treatment programme.

I suggest that attempts at intercourse continue to

be put off for a further four weeks. For those of you who have gone through Stage I this may seem a bit much, but when you think about what you stand to gain it is worth the effort. If either of you desire orgasm this can be achieved by alternative methods already mentioned.

Now, are you able to comfortably insert tampons? If yes, go on to the next step, if no, this is where we begin. Every day, even when you are not menstruating, I want you to practise inserting tampons.

Sit normally on the toilet with your legs apart — if you try doing this on a normal chair it will mean your vagina is squashed flat, making insertion rather awkward. Next, put plenty of K-Y Jelly, Lubafax Gel, or baby oil around the vagina, and, if possible, a little inside. Some women prefer lanolin at this stage which, although greasy, gives a thicker covering of the vagina.

Next, choose a tampon without a cardboard applicator, and rub some oil on its tip.

Then, tighten your vaginal muscles as much as possible, as you have learnt to do from the exercises. Lean forward and place the tip of the tampon against the vaginal opening, which you are still tensing as much as you can. Now, as you slowly let go of that tension, gently push the tampon forward. You may even find it easier if you bear down, that is, as if you are pushing something *out* of your vagina. This can help the vaginal mouth to open more easily. *Do not* push to the point of pain, but mild discomfort is to be expected. Even if you only manage to insert the tampon one millimetre you have done well and are on the road to success.

This should be practised daily until you can insert the tampon easily. If you wear a tampon during menstruation and it feels uncomfortable, you have not pushed it in far enough past the muscle ring at the vaginal entrance (Chapter 2). When you try to get the tampon out, again relax the muscles before doing so. Once the flow decreases, you would be advised to use pads, as the tampon dries the vagina making it slightly more difficult to get it out. This is easy for non-vaginismic women to cope with, but you need to avoid unnecessary discomfort for the time being.

Some women find the tampons awkward and prefer to practise with their fingers. Because fingers are not absorbent, it is easier to make them very slippery with oil or lanolin. You may prefer to wear surgical gloves which can be purchased from a pharmacy. Follow the same procedure as with the tampons, starting with your little finger. Then use your index finger and, when you can comfortably insert that one, try with your middle finger. But proceed at your own pace. It may take a month just to be able to insert your little finger, or it may only take a few attempts.

It is also useful if you can acquire a set of vaginal dilators once you can successfully insert a tampon, or your index finger. Vaginal dilators look somewhat like test-tubes but, as the name implies, they are designed specifically for vaginal use. There are six in a set, ranging in diameter from about the size of a 10-

cent piece to one that is about the size of an erect penis. Ask your doctor if he can help you purchase them, or contact a medical supplier.

You can practise over the toilet, or, at this stage, choose a time when you are going to be alone and uninterrupted and use the bedroom. Get several pillows and arrange them so that you are in a half-sitting position, while still being comfortably supported. Bend your legs and put lots of lubrication on your vagina and the dilator. As before, tighten your vaginal muscles and, as you let go, *gently* insert the dilator. Again, do not push to the point of pain but try to cope with mild discomfort.

When you can comfortably insert one, go to the next size up. When you can comfortably insert size six, it is time to bring your partner in on this part of the programme.

First of all, he must agree to be guided by what *you* can cope with. He needs to be very patient because it can be hard for him to understand why he simply cannot push the dilator in quickly.

Lie on the bed as before and have your partner sit comfortably, where he has easy access to your vagina. Make sure you are supported by pillows because if you strain you are going to be making your vagina tense. Use lubrication as before and start with the smallest dilator.

He holds it in his hand and you hold and guide him. You are the one, at this stage, to move his hand. Do everything as you did on your own, it is just that his hand is holding the dilator as well.

When you have been able to work your way through all six dilators (however long that takes:

days, weeks or months; go at *your* pace), he then does it on his own, but still being guided by your instructions.

Next, when this is accomplished, he does it on his own without instruction.

Once this has been achieved, you are ready to try intercourse. Again, make sure you are comfortable, put some pillows under your backside, or even lie with your bottom on the edge of the bed, him kneeling on the floor and your feet supported by stools or chairs.

Always use a lubrication, both on the vagina and on his penis. Experiment with different types of lubrication such as K-Y Jelly, lanolin, hand cream, baby oil, or vaseline and see which you prefer.

Now, there is a problem here. It is *very* difficult for your partner to produce an erection on demand and, if you just concentrate on entry, you can make yourself very tense. Therefore, I suggest that before any attempt at intercourse is made, you spend some time on foreplay, relaxing, cuddling and touching. However, you might be advised to avoid attempts at arousal and orgasm, as one aspect of arousal is increased muscle tension of the pelvic region.

It may help the man to remain aroused, as well as give you confidence, if you hold his penis when intercourse is attempted and guide it into the vagina. Remember to tighten the vagina as tight as possible just prior to entry, then relax as it is inserted.

At first attempt, to the great frustration of both of you, the penis may only go in one centimetre. But once the woman experiences pain, you must stop and try again another time. Do not just give up in tears but try to support and encourage each other, even though you both may be feeling very diasppointed and even, perhaps, angry. If either of you feel the need for orgasm, alternative methods can be used.

Though progress may be slow, try not to become too discouraged. You are not silly, neurotic or frigid. Just take your time and don't push yourself to the point of pain, but at the same time try to cope with mild discomfort. Try to practise a couple of times a week; you will not make any progress if you avoid attempts at sex altogether.

By following this step-by-step approach, it is highly likely that your vaginismus will be overcome. But it takes courage, patience and understanding. At times one or both of you may feel like giving up, but try to talk it out, and continue with the programme.

PAINFUL INTERCOURSE

In this section I am referring to the woman who can permit the penis to enter the vagina but usually, or always, experiences pain when this takes place.

Compared to vaginismus, there is more likelihood that this condition has a physical basis.

The essential first step in determining what is the cause of the pain is an accurate, detailed description of what the pain feels like, where it occurs and under what circumstances, when it began, and whether the pain occurs at times other than intercourse.

It is also essential that a very thorough medical examination be done. It is not enough for your doctor merely to feel into the vagina with her fingers, or worse, with a speculum, and then decide your problem is emotional. There are at least 20 different medical conditions which can be associated with painful intercourse. Unfortunately, these seem to be overlooked all too often.

Therefore, you need to do some detective work on your own before you arrange an appointment with your doctor. It will clarify the problem if you answer the following questions and take the information with you.

1. *When did you first experience the pain?*
2. *Has the pain changed since that time?*
3. *Is the pain at the opening of the vagina, or deep inside?*
4. *Is there more than one type of pain; for example, when your partner first enters, then deep inside?*
5. *Does it make any difference whether he thrusts slowly or quickly?*
6. *Does it feel as if he is hitting something?*
7. *Can you locate the pain in exactly the same spot every time, or does it occur in different places?*
8. *Is the pain as he enters, or during intercourse, or after intercourse?*
9. *If your partner (gently!) puts his finger in your vagina, can you guide him to the tender spot? Can he feel a hard spot, or a lump?*
10. *Does it only happen in certain positions during sex?*
11. *Do you lubricate, or are you usually dry, when you try intercourse?*

12. *Do you experience the same pain at any time other than intercourse?*
13. *What does the pain feel like: burning, raw, sharp, a dull ache?*

If the pain you feel is at the mouth of the vagina, is not always in exactly the same spot, and you do not usually lubricate, then it is highly likely the pain is caused by anxiety. This anxiety is similar to the fear of pain experienced by the vaginismic woman discussed in the last section. It is not mysterious and complicated, so do not make yourself worse by telling yourself you are frigid and neurotic. Such anxiety usually develops for a good reason and, if the exercises suggested here do not help, please do not be too embarrassed to see a qualified counsellor.

If the pain is inside the vagina, is always in the same spot, particularly when it is on only one side of the vagina, if it feels like your partner is hitting something tender and/or if you experience this pain at times other than during intercourse, it is very probably physical in origin. Another pointer is if you lubricate adequately but still feel pain.

Sometimes, having experienced the pain so often in the past, the woman will reach the point where she fails to lubricate because of her realistic fear of pain. Under these circumstances she may well experience two types of pain, one caused by the physical problem, the other during entry due to lack of lubrication and tension of the vaginal muscles.

If the pain is a burning sensation, it may be due to an infection, or it may be caused by the rubbing of the penis on the dry vagina. Sharp pain is more likely to be physical in origin, a feeling of general discomfort possibly anxiety. And so on.

Do not be put off with the idea that it is "all in your head" if you have enough reason to believe that there is a physical cause.

However, if it seems likely that your problem is due to anxiety, here is what I suggest you do.

As with vaginismus, think about how you feel during foreplay. If you cannot relax and enjoy foreplay, talk to your partner about banning intercourse for a month while you learn to appreciate being held and cuddled. Try also to get your mind thinking sexually, rather than dwelling on possible pain. Shut your eyes and conjure up a sexual fantasy, or, if that is too hard, think to yourself, "That feels nice, that feels good" as your partner cuddles and caresses you. Do not worry too much about arousal, relaxation is more important at this stage.

Your tension, lack of lubrication, and consequent pain may also be due to poor communication with your partner, so that the wrong things are being done during the lead up to intercourse. As we have seen many times by now in this book, many of the techniques suggested by sex manuals often annoy women, making them irritable and tense rather than relaxed and aroused. If this is the case you may find it helpful to re-read Chapter 4.

Chronic fatigue, disharmony in your relationship and financial problems can all contribute to the problem. Think about what is happening in your life, particularly at the time the problem first began. Did you at that time, or now, usually feel tense, worried, hassled, uptight, tired? If so, this is very likely to be a major cause of your tension and pain during intercourse. If there is marital conflict, it would be worthwhile working on those difficulties before you try to tackle the sexual problem.

Although, unlike the vaginismic woman, you are able to permit the penis to enter your vagina, it still may be worthwhile following the programme set out in the previous section. Practise the vaginal exercises on page 195 and use them in the same way as the vaginismic lady, when you are trying to insert the dilators or attempting intercourse. By practising with the dilators, you will reassure yourself that your vagina can accommodate a penis without pain. Talk to your partner about your fears and ask him to cooperate by following your instructions when intercourse is attempted. During intercourse, try to speak calmly to him, asking him to move more slowly, or move his body with your hands, or whatever you need to do in order to feel more in control of the situation and experience less discomfort. *Always* use a lubrication if you are dry.

If you experience great discomfort, stop. However, try to tolerate and, more importantly, ignore mild discomfort by shifting your mind to thoughts such as how nice his body feels close to yours, or by having a sexual fantasy, or anything that acts as a distraction. You need to learn to relax discomfort away. If you feel discomfort when the penis is inside, try the vaginal exercise: tighten your vagina as much as you can, then let go. This will feel nice to your partner as well as helping you reduce the muscle tension.

If you stop because of discomfort, do not just

roll over and go to sleep. Cuddle your partner, comfort each other. If either one, or both, of you desire orgasm, try alternative methods already discussed. Avoid ending everything in anger or frustration, as this will only make future attempts at sex more stressful.

In some cases there are physical causes to the pain that do not warrant or permit medical intervention. Some women with a retroverted uterus (that is, a womb tilted backwards instead of lying forward in the normal position, as in Figure 2), for example, can experience pain with deep, sudden penetration. In these instances the couple need to experiment with different positions to find one that does not cause pain. Again, the woman might need to regularly use vaginal lubrication. By experimenting together you should come up with some suitable alternatives to the more traditional, but painful, methods of intercourse. It may be worthwhile purchasing a book on different sexual positions to give you some ideas.

Vaginismus and painful intercourse are both distressing problems to cope with. Try to keep in mind that as you and your partner cooperate to overcome the difficulty, you are strengthening your relationship and may in the end develop a very secure, comfortable, trusting relationship that more than compensates you for your current dilemma.

7 PROBLEMS WITH ORGASM

We have already seen that orgasm is not the be all and end all for women's satisfaction. Nevertheless, it is a nice experience and, not unreasonably, many women who cannot orgasm would like to be able to do so.

Perhaps surprisingly, some men also have problems with orgasm. I am making the distinction here between ejaculation, which is the physical action of expelling semen, and orgasm, which is the enjoyable experience of that physical occurrence. We have already discussed problems with ejaculation; yet some men can ejaculate but fail to enjoy it, and this needs to be dealt with.

FEMALE ORGASMIC DIFFICULTIES

How do you know if you are having an orgasm?

It is important to be clear about what an orgasm is, so that you know what you are aiming for. I mentioned in Chapter 2 that I disagreed with the widely held belief that if a woman is unsure about whether she has an orgasm, then she probably hasn't.

This confusion a woman (and her partner) may

feel about whether or not she can orgasm arises from the fact that orgasm is usually described in superlative terms. The notion that there are many types of orgasm does not seem to have been given much emphasis.

Perhaps the best way to clear up this confusion is to compare an orgasm to a sneeze, since they are similar in many ways.

The first phase in the development of a sneeze is when the nose is stimulated in some way. This may be by dust, sunlight, pollen and so on. The nose begins to feel congested and the muscles around the nose start to tense.

At some point, a sneeze occurs, but depending on the amount and type of stimulation, the sneeze may be a sudden explosive effort causing people in the room to jump, it may be a minor, quiet little effort which goes largely unnoticed, or, usually, it is the type that falls somewhere in between. All of these are considered sneezes, none is considered abnormal.

Sometimes, however, the build-up in stimulation does not end in a sneeze. The person may be distracted or, for some other reason, "misses" the sneeze and the nose remains congested and irritated. On other occasions, despite early promise, the sneeze just fizzles out without any remaining irritation.

Just so with orgasm!

If you are trying to decide whether you have ever had an orgasm, do not look for the equivalent of the room-clearing sneeze.

Think about what you feel, either during foreplay or intercourse. Do you get a pleasant physical sensation, a bit of a buzz around the vulval area? Does it seem to build, even slightly, and afterwards you feel kind of relaxed, cuddly and sleepy? If so, *this* is an orgasm, even if it is the mini-variety.

You do *not* have to be aware of a pounding heart, feel hot, be writhing in ecstasy, yell out in delight, grimace with glee or any of the other things that have been used to described orgasm. These *may* happen, certainly with the top-of-the-range type, but they are not essential.

Also, the man may be completely unaware that his partner has had an orgasm. A woman I saw recently said she did not orgasm because her partner said he never felt anything. However, she did get this nice trembly feeling . . .

While sex researchers Masters and Johnson say that the vaginal walls contract during orgasm, and while in some instances a man may feel pressure on his penis when his partner comes to orgasm, the fact that the male does not feel this is no indicator of the woman's response.

If you now realise that you are already having at least mini-orgasms, then you may well find that merely by relaxing and enjoying the sensations you already experience, over time your orgasmic ability will improve. One of the main reasons why some women fail to recognise and appreciate these orgasms is that they are so busy concentrating on what should or might happen that they are squashing the sensations they are actually having. Sex becomes hard work rather than a relaxed appreciation of whatever is going on, and we have already seen that tension or worry decreases a woman's arousal.

However, if you wish to develop your orgasmic

potential in a more active way, you might find the following section helpful.

Suggestions for the development of the orgasmic response

The difficulty in giving suggestions on how to overcome problems with the orgasmic response is that you are all likely to be at different levels of sexual response, and you may be wanting to achieve different things. Some women may be prepared to try the suggestions, others may find them unacceptable. Therefore, what I will do is try to provide as much information as possible by using a series of questions and answers. In this way you can select the questions that are relevant to you, and utilise any of the information that you find acceptable. However, I must point out that orgasm is primarily a learned response; it usually takes practice and patience. It is unlikely to develop automatically, particularly if your background is somewhat conservative or inhibited. If you cannot accept *any* of the suggestions given here, or simply cannot be bothered to persevere with them, then your appreciation of sex will need to focus on the emotional aspects.

1. Why do you want to become orgasmic?

If you wish to do so merely to please your partner, or because you believe you are inadequate if you can't, I fear you may find that you progress very little. Like the man's erection, you cannot make yourself have an orgasm. You can only allow it to happen by enjoying and building on the sensations developed by the right stimulation. Orgasm is a very selfish thing, in some ways, because at the point of orgasm all that you are aware of is the pleasurable feelings within your body. If you are worried about other things, such as what your partner is thinking or whether you are normal or not, you will find it difficult to develop the ability to be splendidly self-centred for that moment of time.

2. Do you, under any circumstances, feel aroused?

Some women who would like to become orgasmic feel they have never experienced any degree of arousal, although they may find sex enjoyable. The first physical sign of arousal in the female is lubrication of the vagina. Therefore, unless the woman is always dry when she has sex, *something* turns her on at least a little. She needs to spend some time thinking about what it is that either happens during foreplay, or she thinks about, that produces that response.

Some women find that reading a book with a sexy scene in it, or watching a movie, gives them a slight buzz. Even a mild reaction is proof that you *can* arouse. You and your partner just need to spend some time looking for whatever it is that is likely to help you feel aroused, even if this means keeping a supply of your favourite books on the bedside table. Reading can be a very suitable form of foreplay for women, because it can combine relaxation with arousal.

For the woman who has never felt aroused, perhaps you are avoiding thinking about, reading about, or watching films that contain sexual scenes. It is not abnormal or perverted to enjoy this and you might find that if you give yourself permission to try, you might get something out of it.

I might add, however, that many women are turned off by sexually explicit or hard-core scenes. They often prefer more subtle descriptions, perhaps the R-rated movie but not the X-rated. Women also seem to prefer to read about a sexy scene rather than watch one in a movie. The idea is to explore some of these possibilities to see what, if anything, does make you feel aroused to some degree.

3. Can you have sexual fantasies?

One of the reasons men can arouse so readily is due to the fact that they can use their minds to increase their arousal. During their adolescence, their practice with masturbation has enabled them to develop sexual fantasies, sometimes of a surprising variety.

For a number of reasons, including the infrequency of female masturbation and the general repression of female sexuality, many women find it extremely difficult to think in an explicitly sexual way. This can be part of the reason why some women find it almost impossible to build up arousal during foreplay or intercourse. Some women think about the most amazing things during sex. What will we have for dinner tonight? I wonder if the kids are warm enough? Has the garbage been taken out?

I would encourage women to develop their ability to think erotically and to have enjoyable sexual fantasies. Being able to think sexually helps you to anticipate sex with pleasure, as well as helping to keep your mind on what is happening rather than wandering on to all sorts of irrelevant topics. You cannot have an orgasm if you are thinking about what you are going to buy at the supermarket tomorrow.

Therefore, once you have read a few books or seen some movies that you find even slightly arousing, try to recall these scenes at other times. You may do this while you are lazing in the bath, during foreplay, while you are masturbating, and so on. You may practise in bed at night, like telling yourself a bedtime story. Your fantasy may include your partner, or it may include other men. Some women feel guilty about fantasising about someone other than their partners. If you really do not believe it is right, make your partner your fantasy man. But fantasising about others is a normal and healthy part of enjoying your sexuality. It does not mean you love your partner less or that you intend to wander, it's just nice to think about.

In the same way, you may find the thought of something like rape exciting in fantasy. This does not mean that you wish to be raped, or that you would enjoy being raped in reality. Sexual fantasies are no different to any other daydream. They are a chance to explore forbidden or unattainable territory with safety. It is surprising how many seemingly conservative people in happy, stable relationships have unusual, even bizarre, sexual fantasies.

If you cannot develop fantasies, you can stop your mind wandering during lovemaking by verbalising, either in your mind or out loud, how you feel about what is happening. For example, you might mentally focus on your partner's hands as they move over your body, and say to yourself, "That feels good, that feels nice, that feels sexy", and so on. Some couples find it quite arousing to talk to each other in this way, and can sometimes become quite uninhibited in their language.

Another technique for keeping your mind on the job and to aid arousal is orgasmic role-playing. This is quite different to faking orgasm. Faking implies that you are deceiving your partner, while you yourself get very little out of sex. With role-playing, you let your partner know what you are doing. Then you writhe and move and sigh *as if* you were becoming aroused. You might start out somewhat conservatively to begin with, but once you get into the swing of it you will find yourself loosening up and becoming aware of your body as a source of sensual pleasure. By role-playing in this way, you learn to let go, to stop rigidly controlling your response. While you may feel silly to start with, this technique has been found to be very useful in helping to break down a woman's inhibitions and to build arousal.

4. What happens during foreplay?

Another reason why the woman's mind wanders during sex is because she has not been given enough time to switch off before attempts are made to arouse her. I have mentioned several times already that women need to feel relaxed before they can become aroused. So, if you launch immediately into breast or genital stimulation without any time to settle down and enjoy being together, you will find yourself continuing to dwell on mundane things. You and your partner need to talk over and experiment with the things that are likely to make you feel comfortable and relaxed, whether it is chatting, having a massage, or whatever, before you try to become aroused.

5. Do you try to relax your body during arousal?

I have just said that you need to feel relaxed before you can become aroused, but there is a paradox here. Part of the orgasmic response is muscle tension. Therefore, the initial stages of foreplay need to be directed towards feeling relaxed, particularly mentally, but if you are becoming aroused it may actually help you to deliberately *tense* your muscles, particularly around the genital area and thighs. Experiment with this and see if it makes any difference for you.

6. Can you tell your partner what you like and do not like, and does he listen?

This is always an essential question in any sexual problem and it is certainly worth repeating. You need to be able to indicate to your partner what you would find arousing. However, I appreciate that it is very difficult for some women to say something as explicit as, "Suck my breast". Perhaps, to begin with, you could indicate your desire by the way you position your body, or by moving his hand, or pulling his head down. Some men may be offended, perhaps, but I think the majority would be delighted. Certainly it gets easier with practice, so start with something easy like, "Kiss me", and gradually build up to the more difficult things. If he doesn't listen or act on what you suggest, you might try to talk about this to find out how *he* feels; he might need a bit of encouragement to overcome some of his own inhibitions.

7. Do you and/or your partner believe you should try to become aroused and reach orgasm during every sexual encounter?

If so, you are setting yourself a very difficult task and one that is very likely a key factor in your current orgasmic difficulties. Only experiment with arousal on those occasions (preferably not late at night) when you are feeling quite relaxed and happy with the world. You now know from what you have read already that for a woman, her time to reach orgasm increases if she is feeling tired, anxious, etcetera. If this is true for a woman who can usually be orgasmic, how much more so for you who are just learning to orgasm? Learn to listen to your body. Don't expect it to perform when it is telling you that attempts at arousal are annoying or irritating. If you do persist in trying to come to orgasm, all this does is confirm your belief that you will *never* reach orgasm, so that next time you try, even if you are feeling all right, you will have to overcome your negative attitude to the whole exercise.

8. Do you get very aroused, but just do not reach orgasm?

Usually this means you are trying too hard. You cannot make yourself have an orgasm, you can only allow it to happen. So, for the next few weeks, you have to decide that you are *not* going to try for orgasm. Instead, you are going to listen to your body and only permit arousing stimulation on those occasions when you feel good. Then, you are going to focus on the enjoyable feeling the stimulation is giving you, whether or not it leads to orgasm. At the moment, by living in the future ("Will I orgasm this time?") you are completely wasting all the enjoyment you could be having with the build-up. During this arousal, practise fantasy and verbalisation. Chances are that you will not orgasm for several weeks using this method so, if you feel frustrated, lie quietly for a while. It takes about 20 minutes for your body to get over that very frustrated feeling that missing an orgasm produces. Gently knead the large lips, or get your partner to do so, to help disperse the congestion.

But *do not* persist with stimulation once you have stopped appreciating what is happening and have started to worry about whether you are going to orgasm, because at that point your chances of coming to orgasm drop markedly.

9. What do you feel when your partner touches your breasts and genitals?

Before I answer this question in detail, you must be prepared to accept one basic assumption. You are not "frigid" so that whatever you feel when you are touched sexually is valid and telling you something sensible about yourself.

If you find breast stimulation annoying, all this usually means is that it is happening too early in foreplay, that you are not relaxed. If breast stimulation is painful, your partner may be too rough, or you may find that your breasts are tender because of premenstrual hormonal influences. Some women enjoy breast stimulation provided the nipple is left alone, at least for a while. At the right time, and with the right type of stimulation, many women find breast stimulation powerfully arousing and a beautiful way to build towards orgasm. For others, however, breast stimulation under any circumstances is a complete turn-off. If that is the case with you, you can try it from time to time, but if you don't like it, there is no reason why you should feel inadequate. People are different, after all, so it is unreasonable to expect that every woman is going to enjoy the same things.

Now we need to consider what you feel when your partner attempts to arouse you by hand stimulation of the vulval area. Many women tell me in despair that they must be frigid because they cannot bear that type of stimulation. But your body is a marvellous creation, not readily given to illogical responses, so let's consider what your responses might mean at a logical level.

If you find clitoral stimulation *annoying/irritating* this means either that it is happening too soon in foreplay, or that it is entirely inappropriate on that occasion. Sometimes genital stimulation is the first thing the man tries, because after all, it is great for him. You need to let him know that it drives you crazy, and that you need some gentle cuddles first. But if your body is tired, tense, sluggish, then give away any idea of genital stimulation on that occasion, as arousal is probably out of the question.

If you find clitoral stimulation *painful*, your partner is probably pressing too hard on the clitoris itself or, again, the stimulation may be premature. Tell him that your clitoris is just as sensitive, perhaps more so, than the head of his penis, or his testicles. He couldn't cope with a lot of pressure on those areas, and neither can your clitoris. Gently does it.

If the stimulation is causing a *burning* sensation,

your vulval area is too dry, and possibly his hands are too rough (does he do a lot of manual work?) The solution is simple: a little bit of baby oil or mild hand cream.

If you get the feeling that it is *too much*, that you are being overstimulated, he is probably touching the clitoris directly, when in fact you would respond better to stimulation around or along the side of the clitoris. Experiment with different methods.

If it feels nice, but then you often *lose it*, usually this means that he starts out doing the right thing, but then changes it in some way. Often this is because he is getting no feedback from you that what he is doing feels good, so he thinks he had better try something else. You need to be very clear, perhaps saying out loud that it feels nice, and letting him know that you do not want the stimulation changed. But sometimes his hand gets tired, so it is inevitable that he will change his hand movements in some way on some occasions. And once you have lost the feeling, it can be impossible to get back. All you can do is accept this with frustrated resignation, and try again next time.

There may be other responses that I have not dealt with here. Think calmly and logically about what is going on and you may well come up with the answer yourself.

10. Have you been able to reach orgasm in the past?

There are several possible reasons why a woman might lose the ability to come to orgasm.

The most obvious one is stress. If you are going through a worrying time, or something is happening in your life that makes you very tired, then quite reasonably your orgasmic ability is going to be affected. If your elderly mother has moved in, or you have a couple of small children, or you are beset by financial worries, don't pressure yourself to try and turn on. If you start to worry about this "sex problem" as well, then even when the stress lessens, your anxiety about your lack of response will mean that you will continue to have orgasmic difficulties.

Sometimes a woman was orgasmic with a previous partner but is not with the current one. This can obviously be a very sensitive topic to deal with. The woman often knows what turned her on with the previous partner but is reluctant to tell her new partner. I suggest a lot of tact, which will mean not comparing him directly to the other fellow, but gently educating him about the things you like. It does not necessarily mean that the first fellow was the better lover, merely that he happened to discover and enjoy some of the things that turned you on. You may find that by starting afresh with your current lover, you can develop other things that turn you on, but it can take time to alter your response in this way. Fantasy is useful here.

Sometimes a woman might find that her enjoyment of sex has lessened because her relationship has changed over time. Sometimes the marital relationship has become strained, but often it is just the sexual relationship that has become routine. Sex happens last thing at night, a quick touch of the breast, and then into it. You and your partner may need to get your priorities in order. Spend some time together, have sex earlier in the evening, explore other things you might like to try, get in a supply of sexy books, start talking to each other about what is happening. Imagine you have just met and are making love for the first time. How would you touch each other? What would you do in foreplay? This fantasy can often give you some ideas to help re-vitalise your sex life.

11. Can you come to orgasm by any means at all?

Some women are able to reach orgasm with masturbation, but not with a partner. Some can only climax with oral stimulation. Others cannot come to orgasm under any circumstances.

For those women who can climax with self-stimulation but not with a partner, the chances are that you have taught yourself to orgasm in one specific way. For example, you may usually masturbate curled up in a ball, or using a pillow to rub between your legs. Therefore, when your partner tries to turn you on, he does nothing like the sort of stimulation you have taught your body to respond to. To change this situation, you need to think about what you must do to climax now, and work out a plan of steps which will gradually change the stimulation to bring you to orgasm. Start with what you can do, and practise masturbation, gradually changing the position of your body, or the way you touch yourself. You are aiming to imitate more and more the type of stimulation which would happen during foreplay with your partner.

One woman I saw habitually masturbated lying on her stomach. When she married, she would reach orgasm by lying on top of her husband and moving backwards and forwards. But when she became pregnant, and her abdomen started to swell, this became impossible. Once the baby was born, she decided to do something about her very restricted pattern of orgasmic response. The first step for her was that she would masturbate on her stomach as before, but with one side slightly elevated by pillows. When she could do that, she added more pillows till she was able to masturbate lying on her side. Then she continued the process till she was able to orgasm while lying on her back. It may take you several months of practice to alter your habitual way of coming to orgasm, but it is worth the effort, as it gives you greater flexibility with your partner.

For the woman who cannot climax at all, or who can only orgasm with oral sex, your best chance of learning to be orgasmic is with self-stimulation. Now, this may not be as simple as it sounds. Although masturbation is discussed openly now, and all health professionals agree that it is a normal and desirable thing to do, it is still unacceptable to individual women (and men). It can be difficult to shake off a couple of decades of conditioning that masturbation is wrong and dirty. So, take it slowly. Some of the women I have seen have taken several months before they have been able to accept the idea of touching themselves. Take your time, don't push yourself too much. If you want to develop the orgasmic response, this is the best way to do it, so try not to abandon the idea too readily.

A lot of manuals that advocate masturbation suggest that the woman get a mirror and examine herself as the first step in the programme. I do not think this is essential, although it can be interesting. I suggest you choose a time when you are not going to be interrupted, and get yourself comfortable on the bed, or couch. Lie on your back, perhaps with some pillows supporting your shoulders and head. Use some hand cream or baby oil, and try to find the clitoris with your fingers (go back to Figure 1 in Chapter 2). Locate the two small lips, then trace them to where they join at the top. Start to rub that area gently, experimenting with what might feel nice.

Now, I warn you. Chances are you are going to feel ridiculous/silly/cold/uncomfortable/embarrassed when you do this the first half a dozen times or so. Let's face it, it's not the sort of thing you would have ever thought *you* would do. So don't panic. At first it might be all you can do to lie there with your pants off, let alone actually touch yourself. Take your time. Try to practise at least three times a week, and go at your own pace. It is unlikely that you will experience any pleasurable sensations for perhaps a couple of sessions and you may take weeks to come to orgasm. You have been unable to orgasm for years, so you are not going to change in a hurry.

Tell your partner what you are doing if you think it appropriate, but it is *your* project, not his. The last thing you need is for him to start questioning you about your progress, so try to let him know that you will tell him where you are up to in your own time. Most men are quite understanding about this, because they want what is best for you.

You might read a sexy book while you are masturbating, or practise fantasy or verbalisation. You must appreciate what is happening each moment and not worry about orgasm, which will only happen when you allow arousal to build, and go with these feelings. You may come close to orgasm often, but not quite make it. This is quite a normal part of progress, although it is very frustrating.

If after several months of persistent practice, you still get nowhere, you might consider using a vibrator. The most suitable are not the penis-shaped ones, but body massagers which have a flat rubber pad for massage of the face. These are readily available through pharmacies and electrical departments of large stores.

Again, find somewhere quiet and comfortable, and experiment with the feelings the vibrator produces. Some women find the vibrator is too strong, so you might find it better if you put one hand over the vulva and play the vibrator on that. Some women prefer to keep their legs closed and use the vibrator on the pubic area. It is up to you to discover what feels nice.

Because the vibrator gives strong stimulation, it is highly likely to produce an orgasm in most women after some practice. However, because it is so powerful, it is difficult to reproduce those sensations with your own hand or that of your partner. For this reason I suggest that you continue to persevere with manual stimulation on some occasions, and only practise with the vibrator every now and then. If you can only come to orgasm with the vibrator, you can lessen your dependency on it by gradually altering how you use it. Start by using the vibrator to arouse yourself, but before you come to orgasm put your fingers under the vibrator and start moving them with the vibrator. Over the next few weeks, gradually introduce your fingers earlier. Then, when you can orgasm easily this way, the next step is to take the vibrator off your fingers just prior to orgasm and try to climax only with manual stimulation. By using this approach of gradually substituting your hand for the vibrator, you can learn to orgasm in a variety of ways. The vibrator is always a useful sex aid but it is certainly more convenient to be able to orgasm without it at times. Sometimes there may not be a power-point handy, or the batteries have run down, and it does seem a shame to have your sex life dictated by such mundane issues!

Once you can bring yourself to orgasm with masturbation, you can then try to introduce what you have learnt into sessions with your partner. During foreplay, when you partner tries to stimulate the clitoris, you can guide him with your own hand or by letting him know what you know feels good. You will find that it will take a lot longer to become aroused and come to orgasm with his hand than when you do it yourself. Just as it took a while for you to respond to masturbation, so it will take some time for you to respond to your partner's stimulation. This may well leave you both feeling disappointed, but try to avoid getting upset about it. Patience and encouragement is the only answer. Once attempts at arousal become annoying, it is pointless going on.

You can also introduce the vibrator into your sessions with your partner. Hold your hand over his on the vibrator and show him how you like to use it. But again, try not to rely on it all the time and continue practising with his hand stimulation.

Even when you can come to orgasm with your partner's stimulation, you might still consider the advantages of masturbation. Masturbation has been shown to be the most efficient way for a woman to come to orgasm. Even with your partner, there are times when his stimulation is not getting very far and it makes sense to take over and do it yourself. Now, this involves some understanding and acceptance by both of you that this is a normal and reasonable thing to do, and some couples will find this difficult. But if you can include it in your sexual repertoire, it gives you greater flexibility in your sex life and can take some of the hassle out of trying to reach orgasm.

Please note, however, that many women do not feel comfortable if their partners actually watch while they masturbate, while others find it a turn-on. When you try it for the first time, you are likely to be overcome with either extreme embarrassment or a fit of the giggles. I suggest that he lie by your side cuddling you while you stimulate yourself rather than him take a seat in the gallery. If you cannot climax on the first try, give it a go another time.

It can also be enjoyable to add manual stimulation during intercourse. This means getting into a position that allows comfortable access to the clitoris. Probably the best position is the pregnancy, or non-demand, position, where you lie on your side, your partner lies behind you, and by interwining your legs the penis can enter the vagina. In this position, it is easy to bring yourself to orgasm in a comfortable and relaxed way. This is the position I recommend when you are both feeling lazy and are really not up to a lot of activity.

Similarly, the vibrator can be used either by your partner or yourself during foreplay, and during intercourse. When used during intercourse, the man also benefits as he can feel the vibrations through the woman. To me the aim of these variations is to take the hassle out of arousal and orgasm, by giving yourself as many different methods as possible so that you can choose the most appropriate according to your mood on any particular occasion.

If you want a more detailed programme for training for orgasm, you might find useful a book by Heiman, LoPiccolo and LoPiccolo: *Becoming Orgasmic* (see Bibliography).

12. Do you get any sensations at all during intercourse?

Some women could be reading a book or counting the roses on the wallpaper pattern for all the sensations they feel during intercourse, while others respond easily and quickly with penile thrusting.

Many women are aware of a mildly pleasurable feeling but would not say they were experiencing orgasm. This issue is often confused when the woman is able to climax with clitoral stimulation. She knows that what she feels during intercourse is nothing like what she feels with foreplay. This does not mean, however, that she is not having a mini-orgasm during intercourse. Women who are able to orgasm with either form of stimulation point out that the orgasm feels quite different depending on the method used. I have found a number of women misreading their vaginal responses because they are expecting the same feelings as from direct clitoral stimulation.

Intercourse is the least efficient way for a woman to come to orgasm, so often the build-up in arousal is more subtle. From all accounts the orgasm is experienced as more diffuse, or widespread. That is, with clitoral stimulation strong feeling often occurs in the vulval region, but with intercourse women describe the feeling as "deeper", "spreading all over". Some women may prefer one type of orgasm to the other, while other women appreciate both.

If you would like to improve your response during intercourse, one way is to tone up your vaginal muscles by practising the exercises mentioned for vaginismus and given on page 195. The originator of these exercises, Dr Kegel, found as long ago as the 1950s that regular practice with these exercises produced an improved response for many women within three to six months.

You might also consider the positions you use during intercourse. Bear in mind the new research on the Grafenberg spot mentioned in Chapter 2, and try positions involving rear entry. Even if the Grafenberg spot does not exist, the front wall of the vagina is usually more sensitive to stimulation. Therefore, any position which puts pressure on the front wall may be more arousing. But many find other positions more satisfying, such as the woman-on-top position. The traditional man-on-top position leaves some women feeling suffocated but, by adding a few pillows under the backside, sometimes better friction is achieved. It might be worthwhile getting hold of a book that gives you some ideas about the variety of positions possible. However, a sense of humour is essential for some of them, so do not take the exercise too seriously.

The exercise mentioned in the last section, that is, adding manual stimulation during intercourse, can be used as a bridging step between masturbation and intercourse. The theory behind this is that you learn to associate arousal and orgasm with intercourse by using hand stimulation as well. Once the response is established, you decrease the time used for hand stimulation. Firstly, stop the hand stimulation just as you begin to reach orgasm; then, when you develop a good response to this, stop just prior to orgasm; next, when you are feeling very aroused; and so on. Over a few weeks or months you should gradually reach the point where you do not need extra stimulation at all. Orgasmic role-playing, fantasy, and verbalisation would all be helpful for you to develop your response with intercourse.

MALE ORGASMIC DIFFICULTIES

Most men notice that the quality of their orgasm during ejaculation varies from time to time, and this is quite normal. However, for some, ejaculation produces little or no pleasure most of the time.

The men that I have seen with this problem have all experienced pleasure with ejaculation at some stage previously. However, it is entirely possible that there are some men who have never found ejaculation pleasurable.

I would think that men who have never experienced orgasm are probably similar in many ways to the male with retarded ejaculation. Therefore, if this is your problem you may benefit by reading that section.

The men I have seen, however, have been those for whom sex has become work rather than pleasure. In one instance, the man's partner had a higher sex drive than he, so that he was trying to achieve arousal at a frequency higher than his sex drive indicated. The problem here is the emphasis on penile penetration of the vagina as the criterion that sex has occurred. In this instance it was suggested that if the wife wanted sex when he was not interested, then she could consider self-stimulation, the vibrator, or manual stimulation by her husband. Implicit in this suggestion is the notion that the man is in no way inadequate because his sex drive is lower than that of his wife.

In another instance, the marriage was strained but the sexual relationship continued because of the physical needs of both partners. The man was able to become aroused and ejaculate, but the unhappiness of the marital conflict affected his appreciation of ejaculation. The only solution was to try to resolve the marital problems.

In the few other cases there has been a problem of some ongoing stress, so that the man's sex drive has been depressed somewhat but he has still been able to become aroused and ejaculate with reasonable frequency. Sex becomes an extension of the daily hassles. The man is frequently preoccupied and sex is routine. Again, the stress needs to be dealt with, but also the emphasis during a sexual session needs to shift from arousal to relaxation. Time needs to be spent on talking, cuddles, massage, and intercourse should be ignored unless the man feels refreshed and aroused.

In general, male orgasmic difficulties are less common than other sexual problems. Therefore, there is not as much information available on causes and treatment. This is not terribly helpful to you if this is your problem, but you may find the sections on ejaculation problems, as well as female orgasmic difficulties, give you some ideas on how to overcome your problem.

8 PROBLEMS WITH ENJOYMENT

We all know that sex is supposed to be enjoyable, at least most of the time. At the present time in our society we tend to regard sexual technique as being more important to sexual enjoyment than emotional aspects of the relationship. However, there is more to the enjoyment of sex than knowing what part goes where, or what variations to try.

In the preceding chapters I have discussed specific sexual problems and it is certainly true that such difficulties can lessen a couple's enjoyment of sex. On several occasions, however, I have also pointed out that conflicts or tension within a relationship can seriously disrupt the sexual relationship.

There are other relationship factors which can also contribute to problems with enjoyment or appreciation of a sexual relationship.

1. Commitment to the relationship

Some couples enter into their relationship with the attitude that if it doesn't work out they can split up or get a divorce. Others may have been together for a long time and one or both has lost interest and wants out.

Part of the enjoyment of sex is that you are being close, intimate with someone you regard as special. If your partner is someone whom you wouldn't really care whether he or she was still around next week or next month, then it should come as no surprise that you are not getting as much out of sex as you could.

On the other hand, many of the couples I have seen with sexual problems do have a commitment to one another, but they have not really given it a lot of thought in recent months or years. They have taken their relationship for granted and treat each other as part of the furniture around the place. These couples are slowly drifting apart, although they still care about each other. This lack of closeness will interfere with their sexual enjoyment. The gap gets wider and often the relationship ends.

Give some thought to how important your relationship is to you. If you do not want it to end, now is the time to do something about it.

2. Unrealistic expectations of the relationship

I believe we have been as misled about relationships as we have been about sex.

We watch films and television programs where the characters are involved in relationships that are exciting, dramatic, intense. Happy relationships occur easily because two people are deeply in love. When conflicts occur, they are rarely depicted as trivial (whose turn to bath the kids?) but as major traumas that emphasise the tragedy of love blighted by fate. Everything, good and bad, is larger than life.

But *we* have to come to terms with the reality. Not enough money, not enough room, he won't do the dishes, she doesn't keep up with the ironing, the kids make a racket and there doesn't seem to be any time together. He has to spend the weekend fixing the car or working overtime; she gets no peace from the demands of the preschooler. Where is the excitement, glamour and drama in all this?

It is easy to get disillusioned with your relationship. But, just as we did with sex, we have to put things in perspective. Maybe it would be nice to have more money and lead the glamorous life. But in yearning after this, we can miss out on the wonderful things that are within our reach.

Taking some time off to sit in the sunshine and watch the children play; having a picnic in the local park; cuddling close on a cold and rainy night; sharing thoughts and dreams together; showing you care about each other. These things are important no matter what your lifestyle may be, but somehow we do not take enough time to appreciate them.

And we must also learn to cope with the trivial conflicts that occur in our day-to-day relationships. Few relationships skim along without some friction. Often it is trivial irritations that become the thin end of the wedge in the relationship, as the couple pick and snap at one another. Our grandparents had the right idea when they believed that a good marriage was hard work. A good relationship was two people trying, every day, to get along together and make a good future for themselves. If you are not prepared to make the effort, then you can hardly expect to have a caring and secure relationship.

3. Patterns of communication

One of the most destructive factors in relationship breakdown is the way the couple talk to one another.

We seem to have a major problem in our society.

So many people find it very easy to criticise, and very hard to praise.

It usually starts with the parent and child. The parent always seems to notice when the child does something wrong, but often forgets to comment when the child is behaving properly. Some parents manage to find fault no matter how hard the child has tried. If the parent does praise, it is often because the child has achieved something specific such as doing well at school. What the child needs is unconditional love and spontaneous expressions of that love. Smiles, hugs, kisses, praise, just because the child *is*, for no other reason. This teaches the child that he or she is worthwhile and lovable for himself or herself. Overall, the child needs more positive communication from the parent than negative.

Without this regular reassurance from his parents, the child is likely to grow up believing himself to be inadequate and unlovable. He will lack the confidence to believe that anyone could love him freely (because his parents did not seem to, did they?), and he will not have learnt how to express himself positively to others.

This person, then, may well have difficulty forming relationships with those around him. He or she may form friendships, but have difficulty achieving the closeness or intimacy that is sought. This reinforces the poor self-image and lack of self-confidence that developed during the childhood years.

We see throughout our society people who have learnt to communicate negatively rather than positively. Teacher to student, boss to employee, sales person to customer, friend to friend. And nowhere is this pattern of communication more destructive than between partners in a loving relationship.

Here you are, living with this person presumably for the rest of your life. But where are the feelings of closeness, acceptance and support for each other? Where is the comfort and security? If these feelings are missing, think about how you communicate with one another. Do you find it easier to express negative feelings, that is, irritation, frustration, annoyance, anger, rather than the positive feelings, that is, love, concern, consideration, respect?

Is it easy to say, "You're late", but hard to say, "I'm glad you are home"? Do you criticise, "You haven't taken the garbage out/mowed the lawn/tidied up/cooked tea", but forget to say, "Thanks, love", "You've done a good job of that", "Good dinner", and so on?

How often do you say to each other, "I love you", "I'm glad I married you", "You are still the best-looking man/woman in town", "That was a lovely evening, darling". When was the last time you smiled at one another, shared a joke together, had a good laugh?

Rather than supposedly being confined to the honeymoon stage of a relationship, this positive side of communication becomes more important the longer you stay together. Conflicts and disagreements are inevitable in any relationship and the warm feelings generated by happy, positive communication act as a buffer against the effects of the angry word or the irritated comment.

Even without major disagreements, if you never

say anything nice to one another, how can you feel close? Where is that special feeling that makes you feel like a couple instead of two people who share a house and occasionally have sex? It is easy to forget how much you mean to one another if you rarely express your feelings to each other.

If you do not feel close and companionable on a day-to-day basis, this must inevitably interfere with how comfortable and relaxed you feel when you are having sex. If you have spent the evening picking on one another, you are hardly in the mood to appreciate the joy of being together. And if you carry over your pattern of negative communication into your sex life, you are well on the way to disaster. "Leave me alone", "I don't like that", "You are frigid", "You are a sex maniac", "Do you have to just lie there?", "Hurry up, can't you". What about, "That feels nice", "I like it this way", "No, don't touch me there, I like to just cuddle you", "Hmm, that was nice".

By communicating positively you are improving your sex life because you are teaching each other what you do like rather than just eliminating what you do not. In addition, however, you are making each other feel confident as a sex partner, helping you to feel relaxed and comfortable with one another. It becomes pleasurable to have sex not only for physical satisfaction but for the emotional satisfaction that feeling accepted and loved can bring.

If you have just started to realise that your relationship is dominated by a negative pattern of communication, don't despair. It is possible to develop your communication style slowly, and so improve your relationship. Start with small steps. Say "hello" to one another when you meet at the end of the day, make a point of kissing each other, or having a quick hug, when you leave each other in the morning. Start saying, "Thanks", when you do little things for each other. How about taking him a cold drink when he is mowing the lawn or making her a cup of coffee once the kids are in bed. Build up to, "I'm glad you're home", "You look lovely/ handsome tonight", "You've done a good job on that". Do not be insincere; you are not pretending or making things up. You are learning to express the positive feelings that are already there. When you feel something nice, say it. It can become very easy to smile and say, "I love you", out of the blue while you are helping with the dishes. It is wonderful to be able to say, "I need a cuddle", and know that you will receive the acceptance and comfort you need.

Surprisingly, if you start to introduce the positive aspects of communication into your relationship, in time your partner is very likely going to follow suit without you specifically telling him/her what you are doing. You know how nice it feels when someone praises you, or makes you feel wanted, needed and cared for. This is how you can make your partner feel, and in time he or she is likely to respond to that. Don't give up too easily. If you persevere, you have a lot to gain.

4. Time spent together

You would think that it should be a self-evident truth that no relationship can survive without time being spent together. Yet so many couples I see with sexual and marital problems spend very little time alone, relaxing and chatting.

The children are always around, there is always something to do, and that bane of modern society, the television, is always on. Television has got to be one of the main factors in the current upsurge in marriage and relationship breakdown. Why? Because couples don't talk to each other any more, and how can you have a caring, intimate relationship with someone you rarely discuss things with? Chit-chat is a vital part of any relationship; it is important to be able to discuss the trivial events of the day and enjoy it because you are interested in the other person. And being able to chat makes it easier to lead into the more serious levels of conversation. It is easier to bring up important relationship issues during a friendly, companionable chat than to suddenly launch into a deep discussion out of the blue. Television inhibits this casual, friendly conversation, and ultimately this must affect how close and comfortable you feel with one another.

Television also affects your sexual enjoyment more directly because it means that sex is not thought of till late at night. After all, you can't miss that football replay, or the latest episode of a television serial. Yet, as we have found out in other chapters, late at night is the worst time for a couple to have sex on a regular basis.

Apart from the influence of television, modern couples seem to be caught up in a more hectic lifestyle than our grandparents. Squash, technical college, socialising, and so on, take up many evenings.

This is not a bad thing, in itself, but couples must then make a point of spending some time together. Perhaps you could think of the time after dinner, or after the children have gone to bed, as "our time", when you have a drink or a cup of coffee together and catch up on the day's events.

Try to get some evenings out on your own, as you did when you were courting. Remember how you enjoyed spending time together then, planning for the future or sharing your past? Now, so many couples only ever go out with other people, so they never have those special times together which help you remember why you got together in the first place. If you are not financially well off, a walk along the beach, a drive in the country, or a picnic by the lake, can all revitalise your relationship. You relax together, enjoy each other's company, and rediscover the fact that you actually like each other.

When you spend time together like this, sex is more likely to occur spontaneously as a result of good feeling between the two of you. You are more likely to appreciate the emotional aspects of sex as an extension of feeling relaxed and comfortable with one another, and there is less emphasis on having to perform sexual gymnastics to make sex enjoyable.

A relationship that has little time invested in it is like a flower without water: it will shrivel up and fade away. You must be conscious of the need to plan time together and don't let too long pass between times when you can be together to keep in touch.

5. Coping with arguments

If we were all perfect super-humans who never

made mistakes, were never unreasonable, and were never in a rotten mood then, of course, this section would be unnecessary.

Rightly or wrongly, we are all imperfect, ordinary human beings and so some degree of tension, conflict or argument seems inevitable in most relationships.

We must be realistic and put disagreements in perspective. In a relationship that is basically sound, disagreements should not cause any long-lasting damage. Admittedly for the next few days you might feel a little distant from your partner, and perhaps be a little huffy, but if your relationship is usually characterised by positive communication and good humour, you will almost assuredly get over it. Why? Because you both know that you care for and need each other, and one stupid argument is not enough to destroy what has been so carefully developed over the years.

If you are going to have an argument, there are some basic rules which need to be followed. Always stick to the point of the argument; if you are arguing because someone is two hours late, don't bring in all the other irrelevant issues from past disagreements, like acting disgracefully at cousin Sue's 21st birthday party six months ago. Never, never, say spiteful things to one another because these things continue to hurt long past the end of the argument. How do you take back, "I wish I had never married you" or, "You are a lazy, inconsiderate slob", or worse? If you genuinely mean these things then there is no point in staying together. If you don't mean them, you are obviously saying them only to hurt the other, to get back at your partner for hurting you. Does that make sense? How is that going to help you resolve any problems you may have?

If you do have a legitimate gripe, express clearly why you are angry; you are rejecting the action done, not the person. "I am angry because you are two hours late. Do you think that is reasonable?", "You hurt my feelings when you said that at the party", "I think you did the wrong thing not to help your father", and so on.

Try to persevere until the issue is resolved, or some compromise is reached. Ignoring the issue, sweeping it under the carpet, will only mean that the bitter feelings fester until a future argument brings them pouring out.

Ending an argument may mean that, at least some of the time, it may be *you* who has to say, "I'm sorry". These can sometimes be the hardest words of all to say, but a mature, self-confident person can do it. But, if you are always the one to have to say "sorry", perhaps your partner needs a bit of encouragement to see that it takes two to have an argument.

Some people complain that their partner will never argue with them. This can sometimes be an unhealthy sign. It may mean that important issues are being avoided, or that the partner sees no point in discussing things because she/he wants to make all the decisions. It may be worthwhile reading some books on self-assertion, to give you some ideas on how to assert yourself in your relationship and make it more equal.

There are times when unnecessary arguments develop when they could so easily have been avoided.

If she gets irritable premenstrually, don't add fuel to the fire by lashing back. Make her a cup of coffee, or offer to cook tea, instead. You know it's her hormones acting up, not her. If he has a demanding job, give him time to wind down when he gets home before becoming irritable that he is not helping you prepare dinner. If you both have demanding jobs, try to be flexible about your routine for those times when one or both of you is very tired. If you keep in mind that this is the person you really care about, it is not that hard to brush off the occasional irritated remark or pointed criticism. A smile and a cuddle can be quite disarming, or a sincere, "You're right, love, I'm sorry" ends the matter in one fell swoop.

It is very easy to end relationships today; divorce is common and socially acceptable. But that does not minimise the trauma of separation for the individual. Learning how to cope with and resolve disagreements is a lot easier and less painful than the consequences of heading for the divorce courts when things get rough. Working through relationship difficulties may well mean that you end up with a more secure, comfortable, trusting relationship than you had before.

6. As Grandma said, it takes work

There is no doubt that our attitude to marriage has changed. Marriage is no longer regarded as permanent, as current divorce statistics show. There is the view that the increase in divorce reflects a healthy trend, in so far as it shows that people are now able to disentangle themselves from unhappy, destructive relationships. Maybe it has been unrealistic, in the past, to assume that two people should be able to be happy and contented with each other for their entire adult lives. Perhaps the breakdown of marriage reflects a return to a more normal pattern of behaviour whereby people have a series of relationships rather than being abnormally and artificially bound to a monogamous relationship.

Therefore, the current divorce rate may merely represent a shift in attitudes and behaviour that will ultimately be readily incorporated into the culture. If this is the case, it may be more helpful and productive for counsellors to develop methods of assisting couples to separate without trauma and re-establish the new family units without undue distress, than to concentrate on marital therapy.

Yet, were the marriage partners of a couple of generations ago desperately unhappy, shackled together by restrictive laws? Or were their attitudes to, and expectations of, marriage more realistic, so that they could be contented even though their situation may have been less than perfect?

I think this is an important question to consider because whatever conclusion we come to will shape our attitudes to our own relationships. Certainly, despite the somewhat pessimistic view that the divorce statistics suggest, few people enter into marriage believing that they will end in divorce. Divorce is usually the result of a gradual breakdown of the relationship over time. So what goes wrong between the initial dreams and the beginning of the end?

In this chapter we have looked at a number of possible relationship difficulties that can be a factor in the breakdown of a relationship. I must admit to holding some quite traditional views with regard to commitment to marriage and the concept of the necessity of working hard not only to maintain, but to develop, a relationship. Although our society may ultimately come to terms with divorce, in the meantime, I remain concerned about the unhappiness that is usually generated by marital and long-term relationship breakdown.

Obviously, however, despite what I or anyone else may think, in the end it is up to each couple to decide what sort of relationship they want. Certainly relationships differ from couple to couple without this necessarily implying that there is a problem. If a relationship is based on self-respect, and respect for the other person, then it can be successful whether it is a traditional sex-role type, a dual-career, shared-role type, or any other possible variation. Some couples are less demonstrative, less communicative, and still happy and content. Provided the needs of both partners are being met, they need to have the confidence to maintain their relationship on their own terms.

Problems arise when each partner wants or needs different things from their relationship. In this situation, both partners must firstly recognise that there is a problem, and then be prepared to work together to try to solve their differences. This can only happen if the attempts at reconciliation are based on mutual consideration and respect. Then the couple must work out mutually acceptable goals and compromises.

However, if one partner either will not recognise that there is a problem, or is not prepared to do anything to improve the relationship, then it is extremely difficult for the other partner to do much to salvage the situation. Sometimes, divorce or break-up is the only healthy option available.

7. In conclusion

There is nothing magical or mysterious about a good relationship and an enjoyable sex life. The spirit of this book is cooperation between two people who desire a caring, intimate relationship and are motivated to work to achieve this.

By putting sex in perspective, using common-sense, and by having a sense of commitment to your relationship, you and your partner can achieve the self-confidence needed to develop your sexual relationship to suit yourselves.

9 THE FUTURE

Most books on sex would end there but I have a further concern: what of the adults of the future? What can we, as parents, teach our children so that they are less likely to have the type of problems that are common today?

Sex education is a contentious issue in our society. We disagree about what the youngsters should be told, when and by whom. We also have trouble deciding what is normal and acceptable behaviour from children at different ages.

My own belief is that we are currently handling sex education inappropriately and, unless we revise our current practices, there is likely to be an increase in sexual problems in the future. Films and books are becoming increasingly explicit, but they are doing so in a sensational rather than an educative manner, raising expectations out of all proportion to reality. At the same time, the conservative groups in society are marshalling themselves in an effort to clamp down on sexual knowledge and freedom. Somewhere in all of this our youngsters must be given sensible, straightforward information about sexuality.

In considering this issue, however, we must keep in mind that we are rearing our children to be adults in this particular society and so we need to be aware of what our society currently defines as the limits of acceptable behaviour. While our society has many problems in dealing with sexual issues realistically, nevertheless, there is no point in being completely individualistic about the way you bring up your child if this is going to bring him or her into conflict with the rest of society. This applies, in my opinion, equally to the extremely conservative and extremely liberated viewpoints. I believe we need to change some of our sexual attitudes and behaviours, but we must use a commonsense rather than a confrontationist approach. It is unfair to stand up for our principles at our children's expense.

Before we try to formulate our ideas on sex education, we must ask ourselves a very basic question: what should be achieved by sex education? Obviously, how you answer this question will largely determine *what* you think sex education should be. Some would say that it should teach youngsters self-control, others would say it should lead to a lack of sexual inhibition ("hang-ups", as they say). I believe sex education should provide factual information about the biology of sex, but should not deal with sex in isolation. A person's sexuality is linked with the entire personality and, therefore, sex education should encompass a whole range of issues including self-esteem, interpersonal communication, tolerance of others and so on. I would like to think that we can teach males and females to enjoy being sexual creatures and to be able to make realistic, common-sense judgements about their own sexuality while, at the same time, respecting the rights and beliefs of others.

What follows, then, is a guide to what I believe is a reasonable approach to sex education at various ages. I do not expect everyone to agree with the ideas put forward. But at the very least, I hope those who read this chapter will start to think seriously about this important aspect of our children's development.

I have broken down the ages into three broad categories. There will obviously be some overlap between the groups because children mature at different rates, so in the end it is up to the parents to use their own judgement.

0–6 YEARS

Parents of small children are often worried about their youngsters' sexual curiosity and are concerned to handle the situation correctly. Some are thrown into confusion when little Sally asks, "Where do babies come from?", or Johnny exclaims loudly in the supermarket, "Why is that lady so fat?" Some parents go into great detail to describe the genital apparatus and the process of birth, while others think it is best to distract the child and ignore the issue altogether at this early age.

To start with we must put the issue of sex education into perspective. While we as parents may be anxious about sex and feel uncomfortable talking about it, little children see no difference between asking, "Where do babies come from?" and "Why is there sky?" Their sexual curiosity is a normal extension of their curiosity about life. They are attempting to make sense out of the vast array of concepts, ideas and facts that make up the fabric of their everyday lives. "How can an aeroplane fly?" "Why do cats have fur?" "Why are there traffic lights?" "Why has

Daddy got a penis and you haven't?" "How do you make cars?"

In order to preserve this healthy curiosity and lack of anxiety, the parent ideally should be able to answer one question as calmly and comfortably as the other. If the parent reacts with embarrassment or shame, this may teach the child that sex is something unusual, not a normal part of life.

At the same time, we need to recognise that small children do not require long and detailed explanations of the facts of life. For example, when your child first asks where babies come from, a simple "From Mummy's tummy" will often suffice. Sometime, maybe weeks, later, the child might ask how the baby got to be in Mummy's tummy, and is often satisfied with, "Daddy put it there". Keep your answers simple and to the point. If your child pressures you for more information, it does not mean that he is sexually precocious. It just means that he is curious and his curiosity has not been satisfied. On the other hand, he will often let you know that you have given him more than he wanted by showing disinterest. I remember when my daughter first asked about how the baby gets into the mother's tummy, I told her that Daddy put it there, and then started to talk about "seeds" and the penis. But my daughter reached over to one of her toys and said, "Mummy, when are you going to fix Teddy's arm?" Obviously, she was satisfied without the additional information.

If the conversation gets too deep for you, you could say something like, "It is something big people do, it is a bit hard to explain". After all, can you satisfactorily explain to a young child why there is sky? You are not going to leave your child emotionally scarred if you do not give him adequate explanations for everything. Also, if you feel uncomfortable and embarrassed talking about sex to your children, it is better to say that you will get a book for them to read about it, than struggle on on your own. You are only going to get yourself upset, and give your child the impression he has said something dreadfully wrong. Provided you do not threaten to wash his mouth out with soap when he asks about sexual topics, children are quite resilient and can cope with many different types of response from their parents.

Sometimes our explanations have amusing consequences as the child struggles to digest even the simplest of explanations. My son, at three, wanted to know whether he used to get crumbs on his head when he was in my tummy. This led to one more piece of the puzzle being given to him as I explained about the special place the baby has to himself. The point is that if you can give the information calmly and without embarrassment, your child will explore these ideas with you as they occur to him.

Far more important in the early years is not what you actually tell the child about sex, but what he learns about himself from his family life.

Good sex education actually begins at birth, with the first cuddle from his parents. This is the start of him learning to feel wanted and loved, and to enjoy giving and receiving affection. Over the first few years of his life, the child needs to learn that he is likable, that he is a good kid, and that people, particularly his parents, enjoy having him around (at least most of the time). Learning to value himself as a person is essential for his self-image and sexual development.

It is also the time when you set the pattern of your future relationship with your child. We discussed in the last chapter the importance of positive communication, and this should begin from birth. "Gee I'm glad you are my little boy/girl", "I love cuddling you", "Thank you, darling, you are a big helper". Just as importantly, you need to establish the habit of listening to your child. What is on his mind? Can he talk to you if he is worried? Do you respond if he seems upset? Do you regularly sit down and just talk to him, without letting yourself be distracted by other things?

I am using "he" here simply because it is convenient; there is obviously no difference between the needs of a little boy or a little girl. I have said several times during this book that there are basic biological differences between males and females, which in itself need not be a problem, if these differences are understood. But we greatly exaggerate these differences by the way we bring up girls and boys, and this does seem to lead to problems in adulthood. I would like to see males permitted to be more emotional, females permitted to be more sexual, and in this way both sexes should be able to relate to each other more easily and enjoy any differences between them.

In the early childhood years we make it harder for boys because, despite discussion in recent years, we still often expect little boys to be big and brave, while we feel more comfortable cuddling and soothing little girls. Fathers, particularly, seem to find it harder to cuddle and kiss their sons than their daughters. This puts males at a great disadvantage, for feeling comfortable with themselves and their emotions is an important part of their development into a sexually confident adult.

At this stage we tend to disrupt the sexual development of both males and females by our attitude to masturbation. As you are aware from what you have read so far, I regard masturbation as a healthy and necessary part of a child's sexual development. By telling children that "playing with themselves" is rude and dirty, we are teaching them to see the genitals as dirty. More importantly, we are inhibiting the development of a healthy sex drive and sexual response. This particularly disadvantages females, as we have seen, since unlike males, they tend not to rediscover masturbation at puberty. Therefore, I would like to see our cultural attitudes to masturbation change.

However, this does not mean that we should disregard what is acceptable social behaviour. Just as we toilet-train toddlers, so we can socialise their self-stimulation behaviour. Since children will naturally start to explore their genitals at an early age, I suggest that initially they be allowed to do so without any attempt to stop them. While they are in nappies they get little opportunity to touch their genitals, and from their point of view they are as curious about that part of the body, as they are about their hands, toes, hair and so on. By the time they are out of nappies, you can start to say things like, "I know that feels nice, but it is something you can do in the bedroom or in the bath". At the same time it is quite a simple matter to tell your child that "You don't do it at preschool, or at Nanny's" in a calm way that does not leave the child feeling that there is anything particularly bad or rude about what he or she is doing.

Sex-play between children is a somewhat more difficult issue to cope with. On the one hand we know that it is common for children to play "doctors and nurses", but at the same time it is not acceptable in our society for children to be so obviously sexually curious. In the early childhood years, sex-play is likely to be simple curiosity at what the other sex looks like, and I would be inclined to ignore such behaviour as, for example, looking at each other while bathing or undressing. In fact, this is often the time when questions arise that can be answered quite simply. "What is that?" "That's a penis." "Why does he have a penis?" "Because he is a little boy. Daddy has a penis too. You are a little girl, so you have a vagina/fanny/vulva like Mummy." From my son: "Can I grow up to be a lady like you?" "No, you are a little boy, and boys grow up to be men, like Daddy." And so on.

I would also think that the occasional curious touch to see what the other feels like is acceptable in the early years. However, more intense sex-play can be discouraged by telling the children that you would rather they played another game and, if they would like to know more about their bodies, you will show them pictures in a book (that is, one of the many sex education books available for that age). Although you may not approve of such behaviour, try to remember that from their point of view they are doing nothing wrong. If you overreact and accuse them of being rude, etcetera, you are much more likely to exaggerate their curiosity, or induce feelings of guilt and shame in them.

The same applies to your child seeing you and your partner naked, or making love. Many parents feel quite comfortable being naked in front of the children, while others prefer to dress and bathe in private. My own feeling is that it is quite healthy for children to see their parents naked, to shower together, and so on, but if you feel uneasy doing this, this does not mean your child is going to be disadvantaged in any way. Again, it is more important how you handle the issue, rather than what you actually do. If you do not want the child in with you while you are changing, you can simply say you want to dress in peace. However, if the child accidentally bursts in on you, you can point out that it is bad-mannered not to knock before entering, but try not to get too embarrassed or angry about being caught naked.

While many parents feel that nudity is acceptable, fewer allow their children to see them making love. I think there is a very sound and sensible reason for this: how on earth do you get aroused when you have a small child pestering you for a drink or something to eat! Also, the child may (although not necessarily) misconstrue what you are doing and become concerned that you are fighting. Remember, however, that in other cultures children grow up seeing adults having sex, so this in itself will do no harm. As before, your handling of the situation will determine how your child copes. If you think your child has overheard you having sex and is worried that you were fighting, you can explain that you were playing a game. As the child gets older you can use one of the sex education books to explain that this is what Mummy and Daddy sometimes do, and you prefer to do it in "peace and quiet". If your child catches you unexpectedly, again it is a matter of handling the situation calmly and without embarrassment. Also, if you discover your child trying to simulate intercourse with another child, you can take the opportunity to reinforce the idea that only big people, grown-ups, adults, who care about each other, cuddle each other in this special way.

Generally, if, like most parents, you prefer your child not to see you making love, you can begin to establish rules about privacy. By the time the child is five or six, you can have developed the idea that sometimes Mum and Dad like to be alone, that he or she has plenty of cuddles at other times, and now it is Mummy and Daddy's turn to have a cuddle together.

Whatever your ideas about parental nudity or privacy while having sex, I would encourage you to be openly affectionate with your partner in front of the children. Children usually model themselves on their parents and it is healthy for their emotional development to see their parents hugging, cuddling, kissing, smiling and so on. This encourages them to learn that emotional expression is normal and easy to do. As we saw in the last chapter, this is as important in an adult sexual relationship as knowing the mechanics of intercourse.

6–12 YEARS

Sex education during these years should be a natural progression from the earlier stage.

Masturbation by this stage is likely to be socialised, but if it isn't, persevere with the approach outlined earlier. At this age, you can add more advanced reasoning to encourage your child to masturbate in private. You can say, for example, that just as picking your nose in public isn't the done thing, neither is playing with yourself. While both may be pleasurable, they should be done in private. If your child has his hands down his pants while out shopping, at this age he can cope with, "Remember what I told you about that".

Sex-play may become more explicit and this is less acceptable in the older child, although it may still merely reflect the child's healthy curiosity. If the child seems to be showing excessive preoccupation with his body, or that of the opposite sex, or is frequently peeping through doors or persistently masturbating in public, this may indicate that he has not been given enough information. Some straightforward answers to his questions may be the best approach. In some cases, the child may be behaving in this way to get attention. If this is the case, rather than reacting angrily, it is more important to ask yourself *why* he has this need. Perhaps the child is feeling unappreciated, left out, and if so, this is the most important problem to be dealt with.

At this age, the sex-play itself can be tackled directly. It can be dealt with along the lines of: "I know you are not meaning to do anything wrong, but I would prefer you not to play games like that. Some people might think they are not nice games and I don't want you to get into trouble. If you want to know more about where babies come from, I'll get some books for you and we can read them together. I'll explain anything you want to know."

For the child who is eight or nine or older, you can be even more direct by saying that such behaviour is not permitted and that they should know by now that you do not want them to be doing such silly things. Then, perhaps, you could talk quietly to your child when you are alone at a later time, to make sure he, or she, understands why you are unhappy about him, or her, engaging in this type of behaviour. At the same time you can give your child the opportunity to ask any questions that are on his, or her, mind.

Once children go to school, they may in fact become more self-conscious about issues of modesty, since these values are typically still reinforced at school. Therefore, if your child expresses a desire for privacy, or no longer wants to bathe with a younger sibling, this should be respected. At the same time, they are still likely to accept parental nudity if the parents are quite natural and comfortable about it. If your child makes the observation that other parents don't walk around naked, you can explain that each family likes to do things its own way, and in your family it is all right not to always wear clothes—it is cooler in summer, and so on.

The rules for privacy for all family members can be developed during this age. While the children are little, few parents feel happy about shutting the bedroom door in case the toddler becomes distressed, or gets into mischief. However, the older child can cope with his parents shutting the door for privacy, and the rule of knocking and waiting for permission to enter can be established. This, I might add, should work both ways, where the child has the right to shut his bedroom door. Probably the main reason to set up provisions for your privacy is that as the children get older, they stay up later at night, so that if they become used to their parents spending time in the bedroom you will not have to always delay having sex till after they have gone to bed.

During these years, the child should gradually acquire a sound, basic knowledge of the anatomy of both sexes, and the mechanics of intercourse, pregnancy and birth. Boys should be prepared, by puberty, for the fact that they will one day ejaculate, and what it means. Girls, similarly, should be prepared for menstruation.

As before, however, there is more to sex education than merely giving your child the biological facts of life. During this stage your relationship with your child needs to continue to develop along the lines of spontaneous expression of affection and open, positive communication. Your child needs to feel loved, appreciated, and to know that he or she can approach you when something is on his, or her, mind. You will find that this will become especially important as you enter into the next, and possibly the most difficult, stage, the teenage years.

THE TEENAGE YEARS

Of all the stages of development of your child, the early teenage years are likely to be the most challenging for you as a parent. And I must confess at the outset that I do not have any pat solutions for the parent facing the problems of guiding a child through the teenage years. Sexual attitudes and behaviours are changing so rapidly in our society, at the present time, that at best we can only explore possible solutions.

Twenty years ago, teenagers debated whether they should kiss on the first date. Now the question is, when is it reasonable to have intercourse? It is obvious that more young people are becoming sexually active at an increasingly early age. Some surveys suggest that 70 per cent of teenagers have had intercourse by the age of 19. There is evidence that the pregnancy rate amongst teenagers is dropping because of more widespread use of contraception, but teenage pregnancies continue to occur with alarming frequency. How do we, as parents, feel about this situation? How do we cope with the problems that arise because of it? Do we have any say in, or control over, the sexual activity of our own children?

Before this last question can be answered, we need to put these sexual issues into the wider perspective of adolescence generally. Early sexual experimentation is just one of the many problems that can unsettle the relationship between parents and teenager. Disagreements arise over where the teenager goes, how late he or she stays out, whether he or she smokes or drinks alcohol, as well as issues of dress, tidiness, homework and helping around the house.

For the teenager, the adolescent years are dominated by his attempts to establish his separate, individual identity. No longer a child in his own eyes, he fights for the rights and privileges of an adult. The physical changes the adolescent undergoes are a constant reminder that he is leaving the childhood years behind. Because today's teenagers have much greater exposure to different ideas and lifestyles, particularly through television, they expect more say in their lives than teenagers did a generation ago. As he tries to alter his relationship from one of dependence on his parents to mutual interdependence, the adolescent increasingly questions his parents' values and ideas. The influences of others, particularly his friends, becomes stronger, and his behaviour is often motivated by a desire to be accepted by his friends, even if this brings him into conflict with his parents. He often believes his parents unreasonably treat him like a child, and fail to understand his problems.

The parents' reaction to the teenager's increasing questioning of parental standards of behaviour may be motivated by many factors. Most parents try to instil in their children a particular value system that they regard as correct and appropriate. If the adolescent rejects the parental value system, conflict arises because the parents sincerely believe that the teenager is behaving badly, immorally, immaturely or irresponsibly. Some parents find it hard to accept that their child is maturing and making decisions for himself. Others are concerned about what other people will think if the teenager behaves in a way that is considered unacceptable to the parents' group of friends. But, for the most part, much of the parents' attempt to control the teenager's behaviour is motivated by a natural tendency to protect the child, when the parent feels the teenager is headed for trouble. The parents' attitude to the teenager is often that he is too young to know what is best for himself.

Since the parents and child typically take such contrasting positions on the issues of the teenager's right to do what he wants, it is not surprising that the adolescent years are often a time of upheaval for the family. And, currently, nowhere is this difference more marked than on the issue of teenage sexual behaviour.

In some societies, teenage sexual behaviour is not only accepted but encouraged as a natural, healthy outlet. In others, children are likely to be married and parents themselves at 16. But we live in our society and we must find our own solutions.

Firstly, should we consider early sexual activity a problem? Are we, the older generation, simply overreacting to the behaviour of teenagers, like older generations typically do? Adults are changing their own patterns of sexual behaviour. Premarital sex is now openly accepted by a large part of society and it is common for adults to have sexual relationships with a number of people over a lifetime, instead of the traditional "one and only". Therefore, it should be hardly surprising that teenage sexual behaviour is also changing. Since these changes have already occurred, can we possibly change our society back to more traditional values, and, indeed, should we even try? If there is a problem, what, if anything, should we or can we do about it?

I can only give my personal opinions in answer to these questions, as there is disagreement even amongst professionals about the direction we should be taking.

When I think of my own children, I hope that they will be *at least* 17 or 18 before they begin having sex. I do not want to think that either child will have numerous casual sexual relationships. I do not want them to run the risk of contracting venereal disease, or becoming a parent at a young age. I do not want either child to be used by others who might not care about my child's feelings or well-being.

But the reality seems to be that I have to accept that there is a better than even chance that my children might begin sexual activity at a much younger age than I would like. One of the problems we as parents have is that it is difficult for us to combat the overwhelming influence of the general over-emphasis and sensationalisation of sex which abound in our culture.

So, what are the alternative courses of action available to us as parents?

We can try to influence society at large to present sexuality in a more realistic light. We can campaign to have movies and books reduce the emphasis on sex, and present sexual relationships in a more responsible way. But however much we might want these changes to occur, I think that the current preoccupation with sex is unlikely to diminish in the near future. It is possible that over the next several decades there may be a swing back to more conservative values, because historically, societies tend to go through cyclical swings from conservative to liberal ideas. But this does not help parents of teenagers at this point in our society's development, and indeed, many conservative ideas produce problems of their own, so parents of the future may have a different set of problems to deal with.

At the present time, then, we parents seem to be in a no-win situation. If we disapprove of, and ignore, teenage sexual behaviour, then I believe we run the risk of our children falling headlong into problems out of ignorance. Some parents deal with the situation by putting their daughters on the contraceptive pill, and then pretending nothing is going on. Many teenagers seem to survive quite reasonably under these circumstances, but for me I would like to try to tackle the situation more positively.

But, if we discuss sexual issues openly, without inhibition, are we encouraging teenagers to be more sexually active? I think not, and I'll explain why.

Many parents believe that today's teenagers know all about sex, and are reluctant to discuss sexual matters openly with them. In my experience as a sex educator, today's teenagers may know more about the basic mechanics of sexual intercourse but they are just as confused and ignorant about sexuality as we ever were.

Current sex education is inadequate to counteract the popular sensationalisation of sex. Discussions of contraception, venereal disease, menstruation and birth do little to prepare teenagers to evaluate the conflict between the pressures of society to experiment sexually, and that of parents to avoid sexual activity. Nor does such limited sex education help young people to understand male and female sexuality, and the similarities and differences between the sexes. It does nothing to promote positive acceptance of sexuality combined with a mature ability to make decisions about one's own sexuality. It does not inform our young people about how to conduct an enjoyable sexual relationship, or teach them realistic sexual expectations.

I believe that if we dealt with these issues openly and honestly, we would be much more likely to promote more responsible, mature decisions from our young people about their sexual relationships.

We may still have to accept that early experimentation is likely. But, hopefully, the relationship between parents and teenager has been developed over the years so that the teenager feels confident enough to talk to the parents about any problems confronting him or her. It can be difficult to suddenly try to talk to your child about important issues such as sexuality only when the problems of adolescence develop. However, it is never too late to start talking to your child, and showing him, or her, that you really do care and are trying to understand.

I would like to think that I could talk to my children about responsibility in a sexual relationship, and to encourage them to make decisions based on respect for themselves and others. I would like to be able to support them to resist having sex merely because everyone else does, or because the other partner is pressuring them to do so. But, if they are going to have a sexual relationship, I would also like to be able to give them the information they need to make it a positive, enjoyable experience. I find it difficult to accept the idea that it is all right for teenagers to have sex provided we do not know about it and they do not enjoy it. I am seeing the results of this attitude in the many young couples who now come for sexual counselling. I would like to think that there has to be a more balanced approach which will ensure that our teenagers are given a commonsense, realistic start to their sex lives. Ultimately, this might mean that we accept that our young people are sexually active and permit it to be brought out in the open. Ten years ago few parents could accept the idea of one of their children living in a *de facto* relationship. Now Mother makes up the double bed when the couple come to stay; 10 years ago she would have insisted on them having separate bedrooms. Perhaps, in the future, parents will allow their teenagers to bring home someone with whom they are having an ongoing emotional and sexual relationship to spend the night together.

Whatever direction we take in the future, at the present time our society has failed to come to grips with the changing sexual attitudes and behaviours of today's teenagers. It isn't sufficient to bury our heads in the sand and hope that the problem will go away. I believe that, unless some commonsense is brought to the problem, today's young people will become increasingly confused about realistic sexual expectations, and possibly will be even more likely to develop sexual problems than previous generations.

As I said at the beginning, I cannot claim to have the answers, all I have done is present some ideas for discussion. But I believe that we are failing our teenagers when we avoid tackling the problems confronting them, and then throw up our hands in despair and anger when they make choices which are different to those we would have them make.

APPENDIX

VAGINAL MUSCLE EXERCISES

To identify the relevant muscle group, try stopping your urine flow. Now try contracting the muscle again. You may or may not feel the contractions at first. If you insert a finger into the vagina, you will be able to feel the muscle contracting. These exercises will require some concentration at first, but will become routine after a short time.

The exercises

1. Contract and relax the muscle as quickly as possible, while breathing regularly.
2. Contract the muscle, hold for a count of three, then relax, breathing regularly.
3. Contract the muscle while inhaling, pulling the muscle upward with the intake of breath. This may be harder to do, because you may find your stomach muscles contracting as well. With time you will learn to do this one without contracting the stomach muscles.
4. Bear down on the muscle as if pushing something out of the vagina, or trying to urinate in a hurry. This one is best done before getting out of bed. You may find yourself holding your breath, but try to breathe regularly.

How often?

Find a convenient time *every day* to practise. These exercises become easier to do with time, and only take a few minutes a day.

Exercises 1 and 2 should be done 25 times each, initially, working up to 50 times each during two to three weeks.

Exercises 3 and 4 should be done 10 times each, initially, working up to 25 times each in two to three weeks.

BIBLIOGRAPHY

Chapter 1

Brasch, R. *How Did Sex Begin?* Sydney: Angus & Robertson, 1973.

Malinowski, B. *Sex, Culture and Myth*. London: Mayflower-Dell, 1967.

Tannahill, R. *Sex in History*. London: Hamish Hamilton, 1980.

Walker, K. & Fletcher, P. *Sex and Society*. Middlesex: Penguin Books, 1955.

Chapter 2

Llewellyn-Jones, D. *Everyman*. Oxford: Oxford University Press, 1981.

———. *Everywoman: A Gynaecological Guide for Life*. Second Edition. London: Faber, 1978.

Masters, W., Johnson, V. & Kolodny, R. *Human Sexuality*. Boston: Little, Brown & Co., 1982.

Chapter 3

Haddon, C. *The Limits of Sex*. London: Michael Joseph, 1982.

Simons, J. *Does Sex Make You Feel Guilty?* London: Sphere, 1972.

Chapters 4-8

Heiman, J., LoPiccolo, L. & LoPiccolo, J. *Becoming Orgasmic: A Sexual Growth Program for Women*. Englewood Cliffs, NJ: Prentice Hall, 1976.

Kaplan, H. *The Illustrated Manual of Sex Therapy.* London: Souvenir Press, 1976.

LoPiccolo, J. & LoPiccolo, L. *Handbook of Sex Therapy.* New York: Plenum Press, 1978.

Masters, W. & Johnson, V. *Human Sexual Inadequacy.* Boston: Little, Brown & Co., 1970.

Chapter 9

Knudsen, P. *How a Baby is Made.* London: Pan, 1975.

Llewellyn-Jones, D. *Understanding Sexuality.* Melbourne: Oxford University Press, 1980.

McCarthy, W. (Ed.) *Teaching About Sex. The Australian Experience.* Sydney: George Allen & Unwin Australia, 1983.

Mayle, P. *Where Did I Come From?* London: Macmillan, 1975.

——. *What's Happening to Me?* London: Macmillan, 1976.

INDEX